how to be an Irresistible woman

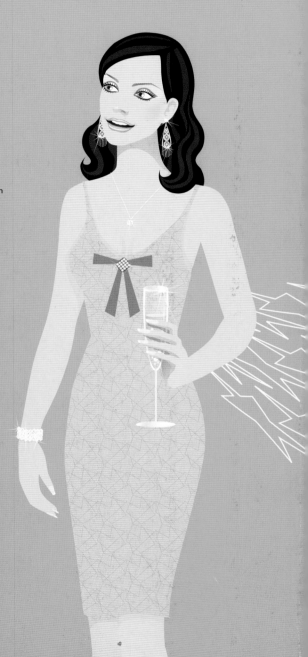

*To my sisters Jo and Suzy, who witness
the highs and lows and are always there
to put the kettle on.*

THIS IS A CARLTON BOOK

Text, design and illustrations © 2006
Carlton Books Limited

This edition published by
Carlton Books Limited 2006
20 Mortimer Street
London W1T 3JW

A CIP catalogue record for this book
is available from the British Library

UK:
ISBN-10 1 84442 251 8
ISBN-13 978 1 84442 251 7

US:
ISBN-10 1 84732 005 8
ISBN-13 978 1 84732 005 6

executive editor: Lisa Dyer
senior art editor: Zoë Dissell
designer: Liz Wiffen
production: Caroline Alberti

Illustrations by Kun-Sung Chung
www.kschung.com

how to be an Irresistible Woman

lisa Helmanis

CARLTON
BOOKS

contents

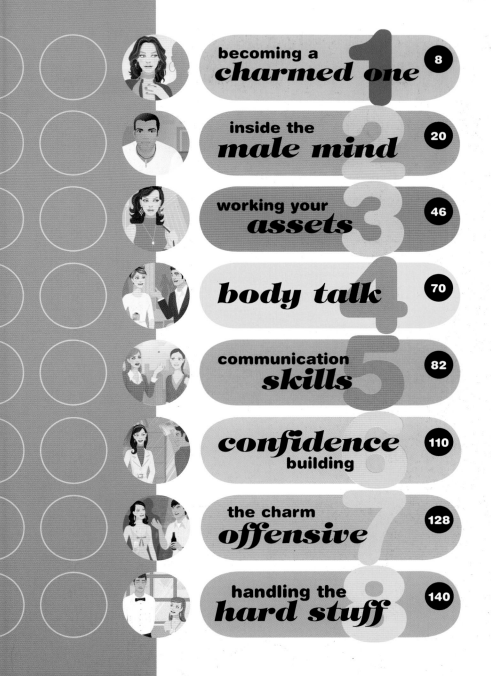

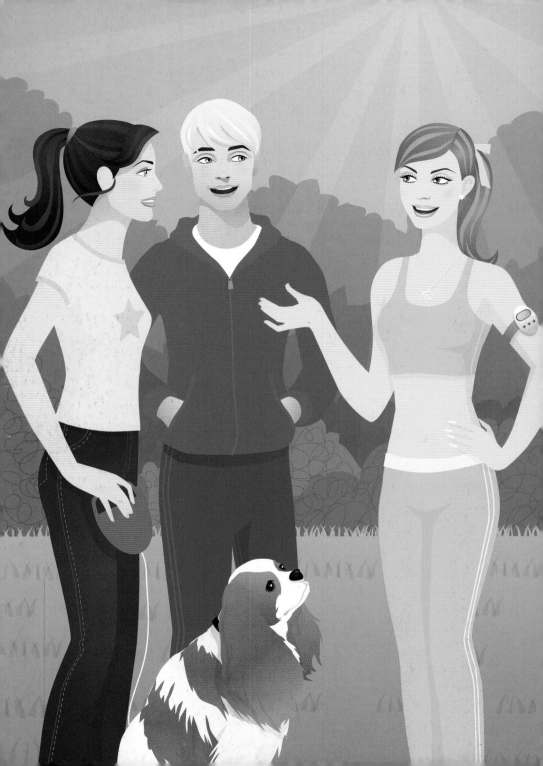

introduction

Everyone knows when a charming person has entered the room. The atmosphere seems more charged, the laughter level increases a few decibels, and even the dullest of dinner parties can seem like the social event of the season. Her attractiveness goes beyond physical looks – she has charisma snd style, and it's effortless.

Charming people make the world a more enjoyable and glittering place, and they are irresistible to most of us who get sucked into their vortex. Time spent in their company is like having the sun turned up a few notches and shone directly onto your face. Having this natural charisma is the most essential component in finding a job, friends and even true love. According to a study by the University of Waterloo in Canada, **85 per cent of men and women rate charm as the main cause of attraction to another person.** Almost all who are like this have irresistible qualities without fully realizing it or knowing why, but these attributes can be learned.

This book will teach you something more valuable than mere acts of persuasion; it will teach you how to be irresistibly charming, not just for others' pleasure, but for your own, too. Life will become more interesting and enjoyable, goals more easily achievable, and success and fulfilment will follow.

When people think of you, do they remember you with a smile, and wonder how they can see you again? Seems unrealistic? It comes down to one simple fact: do you brighten their day?

Win over one person at a time. Start by turning that brief nod to the neighbours into a smiling, life-affirming greeting. You will soon see the powerful impact of this smallest change in attitude.

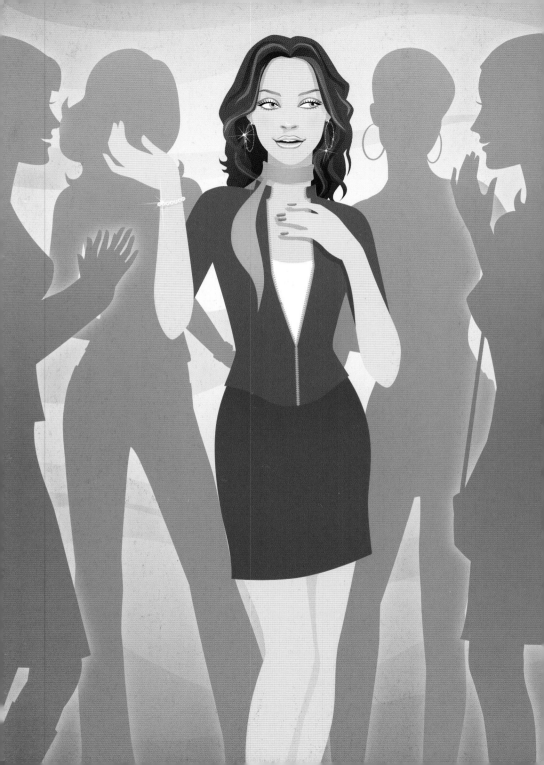

becoming a
charmed one

1

a charmer isn't charming

There is a big difference between being charming and being a charmer, and the first step is knowing the difference. As almost anyone can tell you, a charmer may be seductive but they always come with a health warning. While a charming guest will leave with your guests eating out of the palm of their hand, a charmer is just as likely to leave having palmed the family silver.

A charmer is not sincere; they use charm as a smoke screen to hide their true desires, or simply as a means to an end. (Ask anyone who dated a charmer pre-ceremony, but seems to be married to a slob.) The insincere charmer uses the same 200-watt smile, 'Love your hair' compliment, and nodding head tilt as they glaze over. It's as if they dropped out of Charm 101 after the first term. Their motivation is as likely to be attention-seeking as it is to be manipulative.

The truly charming always tailor their behaviour to the people and circumstances (that tap dancing went down a storm at your cousin's wedding but may not be such a crowd-pleaser at your new boyfriend's uncle's funeral). And the path to becoming a charmed one lies in possessing a genuine interest and curiosity about others that relies on empathy and good manners, not self-interest.

put on *a happy face*

Ever been told that it takes fewer muscles to smile than to frown? Well, that's a lie, but smiling is the speediest route to becoming charming. It actually takes more muscles to smile (about 12 versus 11 for frowning), but it is still easier to perk up your face – human beings smile frequently, leaving those muscles in better shape, so taking less effort to form that grin.

Laughter also has health benefits such as **lowering levels of stress hormones and blood pressure** and relaxing muscles. It also boosts the immune system, improves digestion and speeds up the healing process, plus it makes you thin. OK, so that last bit's not true, but surely all that other great stuff is reason enough to put a smile on your face? And why is it the cornerstone of charm? Paul Ekman, professor of psychology at the University of California, has deduced that humans can pick up a smile from 30 m (100 ft) away; it is a signal to which it is almost impossible not to respond with a similar expression.

When was the last time you found anyone that didn't smile truly charming? You can say all the right things, but without the right expression you may just seem condescending. While learning about the other charming skills, **start smiling at strangers** and see the difference immediately.

first impressions:
make yours count

There's nothing worse than feeling you have to 'recover' from a bad first impression. It can take months to eradicate the impact of an unpleasant or disastrous impression, and even then, the initial impact will always in some way inform their future opinions of you. Scared? You should be.

how they work

Think of your first meeting with anyone as a snapshot they will take away with them. If you are funny, warm and upbeat, even if you display the exact opposite characteristics the next time they meet you, they assume that you are the same cheery person but having a bad day. If they meet you on a bad day when you are harassed and grumpy, they will assume this is your normal disposition, even if you are a joy to behold on your next meeting. This is why the first meeting is essential; it **sets the tone for how they will interpret the rest of your behaviour** from here on in. So if you have managed to put across the qualities you most like in yourself in your first meeting with someone, you never need to regret your behaviour.

how you are perceived

Some friendly people come across as overbearing or attention-grabbing; some shy people come across as standoffish or arrogant. None of this may be true, but as those meeting us don't have a field of reference in which to place our behaviour, we need to be aware of how they might interpret us. **Don't just assume** people see things the way you do. It could be the reason why your mate gets asked out more than you, or why you always end up in the kitchen at parties.

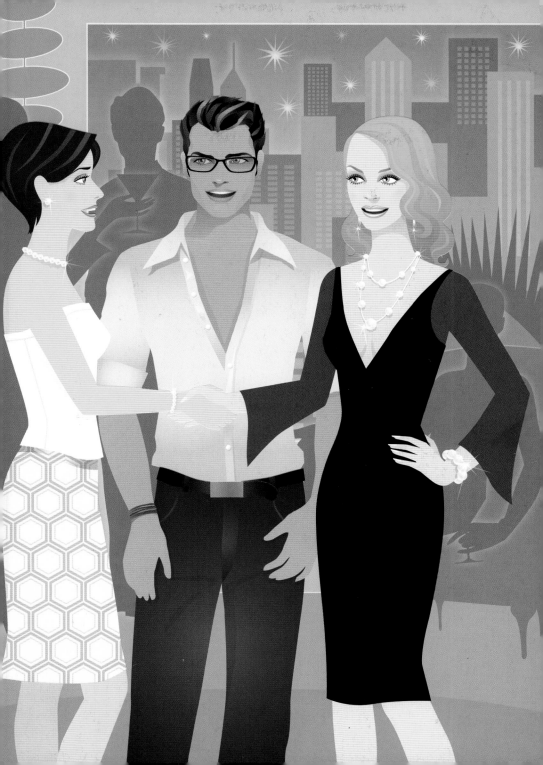

find your
inner celebrity

Make sure you get the body right, too. What makes a celebrity a celebrity? What makes people pause and inhale, turning towards them in wonder? Well, sure, part of it is the fame. After all, it's a highly prized symbol in modern culture. But there is always something else, and if you can master this, you will be one of those people who, when they enter a room, people think: Is she famous? Should I know her? Have I seen her before? I want her to be my friend.

homework

Watch the Oscars and see how the big guns do it. They literally enter, pause and act as though just allowing the audience to gaze upon them is like presenting them with a cool glass of water on a hot day. **They don't demand attention –** they expect it. This is the quiet power you want to emulate. Now watch their interactions. You might find that they rarely interrupt others, as they are confident that their time will come to speak and others will want to hear what they say.

CONFIDENCE IS THE KEY.

show interest and take time to respond

Good listeners encourage the other person to expand on their topics, asking them to elaborate on their initial statements, rather than falling into the classic mistake of saying, 'Oh I know, isn't golf great? I play all the time, in fact this year I went...' Why ask in the first place if you are just using it as a way to wrestle the conversation back to yourself? You may just as well **stay at home with a mirror.**

However, the flip side of talking about yourself too much is to say nothing, leaving your partner casting around desperately for some titbit of info you might reveal and wondering if you are lacking any form of a personal history due to being placed in a Witness Protection Program by the FBI. Basically, a conversation should be an exchange of ideas, thoughts, facts and feel-good vibes. Bear that in mind at all times and you can't go too wrong.

can you really talk about the weather?

Not only can you, you should. There is a reason why weather, bad traffic jams and other seemingly dull subjects make an appearance in our chats with new people. Because we need to do some 'common ground' stuff before we tackle anything more provocative. That's why when you ask someone you just met, or hardly know, how they are, you feel horrified when they say 'The cat died', 'My husband ran off with the woman from the flower shop' or 'I've had such bad stomach bug I haven't slept in days'. It's not that you wouldn't want to share her thoughts on such matters or commiserate with her, but you need to warm up to it: it's like **forgetting the verbal foreplay**, and that just makes the listener feel cheap and used.

' **Brevity is the great**
charm of eloquence. '

Marcus Tuliius Cicero
(106 BC–3 BC), Roman statesman

let them set the pace

Want to know how to never get it wrong? Watch to see how
the other person behaves, **letting them set the pace** when
it comes to talking about personal details and how much they
want to talk. A good model is to split the percentage of time
spent talking by the number of people in the group: so for
two, half the time each; for three, a third each. But some people
like to listen more than talk, so you will need to take up the
slack. (Make sure you are not imposing your preference, ask
yourself if you like to talk more than listen and be aware of when
you need to modify these urges.) In the same way, mimic the
speed of voice. If someone is super-slow, don't literally do an
imitation, but speaking at high speed will probably sound as if
you are screeching at them, even if you are only talking about
eighteenth-century needlepoint. Relax and take it easier.

leave them wanting more

Think about how you make them feel. Everyone has a friend
who leaves them feeling as if they've been **hit by a truck**. Don't
be that friend. If you make someone feel happy, engaged and
inspired, they'll mourn your retreating back as you leave the
room and have a little moment of joyous heart leap when they
hear you'll be dropping by for drinks. But if you leave them
feeling ignored, bored or depleted, they'll turn off all the lights
and pretend they aren't home. If you always want to be greeted
with open arms, aim for the former... Leave them wanting more!

**‘ Always be nice to people
on the way up because
you'll meet them on the way down. ’**

**Wilson Mizner
(1876–1933), US screenwriter**

 16 *becoming a charmed one*

how to *get others to please you*

... and love doing it. This is so easy, it's embarrassing to write. It's so obvious most of us get it wrong; it simply means to make sure they enjoy it, too. You may be able to press gang someone to help you a few times through guilt, pressure or pleading, but the person who's fun, considerate and cracks open the beers for the volunteers who helped them move house will always be able to find a helping hand when the lease is up again.

The fact of the matter is that it's nice to do something for someone; it **makes you feel good.** It makes you feel competent, needed and close to that person, who feels that they are able to call on you, too. A big mistake women make is that they think that asking for help makes them appear needy, or that it inconveniences others. But never asking for help limits the extent of the relationships you have with people and prevents trust from growing. Take a risk – ask for some help and both of you get to enjoy it.

'Charm is a way of **getting the answer yes** without asking a clear question.**'**

Albert Camus
(1913–1960), French philosopher and author

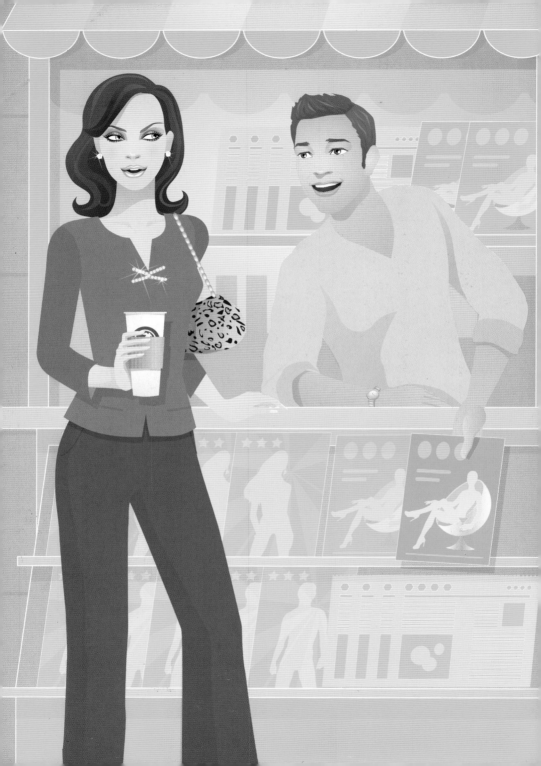

practise your *charm offensive*

Being charming isn't like having a wig; the truly charming don't take it off at night when no one's looking. You don't just save your best self for the guy you fancy at the tennis club. It's a mind-set and, like any new skill, the best way to become a master of it is to practise, practise, practise.

Although it might seem weird at first, once you start getting good reactions, you'll be hooked. Do it to everyone you meet – your mother, dog, friends and even the delivery guy. Not only will this **blanket-bomb approach** improve your day and your repertoire of feel-good anecdotes, but it will help you put any knockbacks into perspective. If the newspaper man is less than receptive, remember he's already been up for hours and there's always the train ticket collector.

the *five* golden *don'ts* of the *charming* woman

During this book you will learn how to make everyone you meet feel great and think you're a real asset to the planet. But while you're learning, make sure you start applying these five golden don'ts to ensure that you aren't making unnecessary enemies along the way. Eradicating these unhelpful strategies from your repertoire will immediately set you firmly on the path to irresistibility.

- ✪ Never leave anyone out. 'Inclusive' is the watchword of the truly charming.
- ✪ Never make a joke at someone else's expense. Tacky, tacky, tacky!
- ✪ Never point out someone's spilt drink, tongue-tied slip-up or drooping hem. Ignore these indiscretions and be loved for it.
- ✪ Never confuse sexuality with charm. Charm, you can use on your old uncle Bob – the other stuff should only be used on him by his wife, Auntie Rose.
- ✪ Never use charm as a trade-off. Charm will open doors for you and ease your social passage, but using it as a bartering tool is just manipulation and emotional blackmail. Put the good stuff out there just because you can.

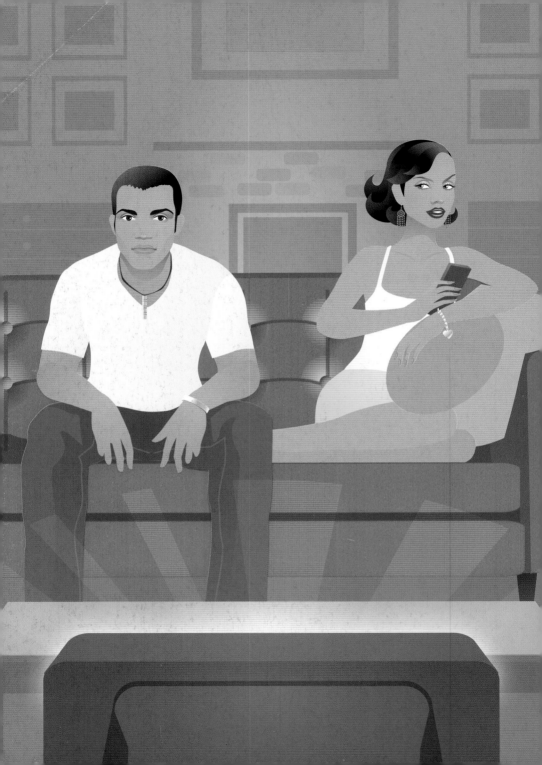

inside the
male mind 2

'An ideal wife is one who remains faithful to you, but tries to be just as charming as if she weren't.'

Sacha Guitry
(1885–1957), French dramatist,
actor and film director

The great thing about being charming is that once you've mastered its arts, you can use it to win over everyone from your gran to your boss (unless your gran *is* your boss, in which case you may be trapped in an episode of *Dynasty*). And all these skills just need tweaking slightly to make you utterly desirable to the men in your life. (These tricks will, of course, work on the girls too, depending upon your preference.)

The great news is that pre-irresistible, you might have felt you needed to work out whether a person was attracted to you before you made your move, but that's the old you. Although you might not be able to win over every heart, you will be able to leave most guys with a smile on their face, thinking, at the very least, 'What a girl!' And research shows that we find people who are attracted to us immediately more appealing. So don't leave it up to him to decide – he simply doesn't know you are irresistible yet.

physical attraction:
how much do looks matter?

Looks matter. They always have and they always will. How a person presents themselves to the world is essential to the success of their progress through it. But the surprising secret about sex appeal is that it has far less to do with our looks than we think.

Research by the University of Central Florida in the US shows that men are more likely to rate a woman as physically appealing if she is friendly and likeable. Did you hear that? **Personality really does count!** So now you know that by being charming you can actually increase your foxiness, how do you harness that appeal? And how do you know when you are doing it right?

‘ Charm is a glow

within a woman that casts a most
becoming light on others. ’

John Mason Brown
(1900–1969), US critic and lecturer

turn up the heat

Think of your sex appeal as a dial with ratings
from one to ten; **you can turn
it up and down** at will.
At work you may choose to
keep it really low (around
a one or two); with a
mixed group of friends
having Sunday lunch
together you may
increase it to a flirty
five; and at a party
where someone
catches your eye
you can kick it up
a notch or two to
a high eight or nine.

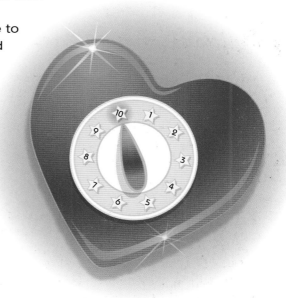

Think through these scenarios and imagine each of your actions (a flash of a smile, a hand on an arm), and realize you can control how hot you are. You do it all the time without even giving it a second thought. So, the next time you are at a party, instead of finding yourself staring at a guy hoping he finds you attractive, remember you are the one who is in control of how appealing you are, not him. Giving it your best shot isn't a guarantee that you are his type, but deciding to **be the chooser,** rather than the chosen, will, at the very least, make you feel a lot more in control of your destiny.

Remember at school when flirting with everyone in the class was as much a part of your day as forgetting your gym kit? When it all didn't matter so much? When it wasn't about finding your true love but making double maths lessons less dull? See flirting as a way of **oiling the social wheels** and staying attuned to those around you – your flirting muscle is like any other: forget to use it, and it atrophies and feels painful every time you try. Flex it every day and you're in fighting shape.

how attraction works:

is there any way in?

Giving men an 'in' is essential. Imagine the scene: the as-yet unrecognized love of your life sees the back of your silhouette in a crowded bar surrounded by friends, drinking champagne and laughing with a man. He is captivated. He comes over, and says, 'I think you are amazing and I want to be with you in an intimate and meaningful way for the rest of our lives.'

NOW, WAKE UP!

Basically, this is never going to happen. **Everything about this situation is wrong.** You have your back to the room so you cannot make encouraging eye contact. He is unsure about the status of the relationship between you and the man you are with. Your friends are an unnerving and possibly humiliating physical and psychological barrier. Your glass is full... Basically he hasn't even got the thinnest of excuses to talk to you. Even if he thinks you are a vision, the only people who start conversations like that shouldn't be drinking with their medication!

making it easy for them to come to you

A lot of women aren't comfortable with the idea of chatting up a guy. So the secret is to **get him to come to you.** Try these subtle ways of letting him know his approach would be well received.

⭐ Regular people need an 'in', even if it's a thinly disguised way of getting to chat you up. An empty glass is a good one.

⭐ The old saying 'if you want to get ahead, get a hat' has a lot of mileage. A point of difference will always help. It may even be as simple as an interesting T-shirt slogan (or a big dog if you're in the park) – anything to give the person a way of having something to talk about.

⭐ If you are with a big group of friends, make sure you go to the bar alone, or move away from the group slightly to chat with one of them, making you much easier to approach. Don't choose the bitter, just-broken-up, heartbroken friend. She may snarl unhelpfully at any man who wants to risk running the gauntlet.

⭐ Leave space for someone to join: don't wedge yourself in a corner or put yourself on the side of the table that's inaccessible to others. If sitting, place your chair at an angle open to the rest of the room.

⭐ Eye contact, eye contact, eye contact… Flick your eyes toward them, gaze, then look down or away. Repeat regularly, making sure you hold their gaze long enough so they don't imagine you are simply trying to read the bar menu over their head. When you have made contact, add a little smile of encouragement. Don't just stare without looking away – it makes you look crazy.

> ❝ There's a **difference between beauty and charm.** A **beautiful** woman is one I notice. A **charming** woman is one who notices me. ❞
>
> **John Erskine**
> **(1879–1951), US educator, musician and novelist**

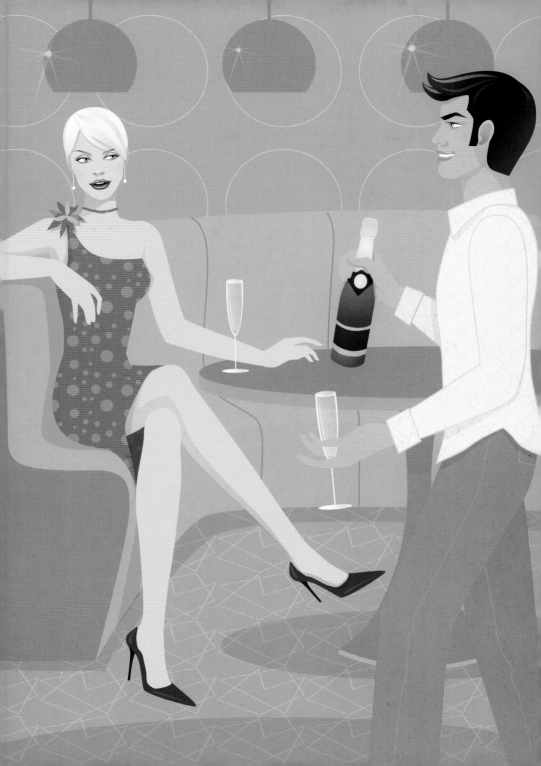

and when he approaches...

- Be gracious. If someone has built up the nerve to head over and make the first move, don't laugh him out of town if his first line is 'Do you come here often?'. He is probably still processing the information that he made it thus far and needs a little time to recover from his rejection anxiety before he relaxes and starts revealing his wonderful witty repartee. If he fumbles or says something stupid, laugh with, not at him. See this as the initial 'contact' phase, not a soul-bearing session.

  - Keep your body angled toward his and 'mirror' his actions (see also page 76).

- If you are interested, make it known. Ask questions, touch his arm occasionally and look into his eyes. There is nothing more enticing than feeling like someone is interested in you. Make sure you let this build as the night wears on. Let him feel as though his fabulous personality is gradually drawing you in. Even if you decided he was fantastic at 50 paces, it makes you both feel as if you've won a prize.

- Never knock a compliment – it makes you both look bad. If he says, 'What a great dress', don't say, 'No way! I got it really cheap because it has a coffee stain on the back and I'm only wearing it 'cos I put on weight and I'm so fat.' Where can you go from there? Try a restrained 'Thanks' and a slow, sexy smile, maybe even returning a feel-good comment.

  - Smile. It's an instant mood-lifter for you both, and encourages him to keep going.

- Keep it clean. Only the very scary or very desperate talk innuendo on the first meeting. If it's a one-night stand you're looking for, then go ahead because that's the message you're sending out. But if you are after anything more, keep it clean. You are telling him by your words and actions who you are right now and, if you act like a bargain basement hooker, he'll treat you like one.

⚙ Show him your best points. Great legs? Get up and walk to the bar or cross them demurely. A bust that deserves saluting? Run your fingers over your décolletage.

⚙ Nothing to say? Talk about something you love – your dog, mountains where you like to go walking... anything that excites you and that you have passion for will show you to be lively and engaged with the world (very attractive qualities) and you will find you easily come up with things to say. Remember, passion breeds passion.

⚙ If you really like him, try this eye-contact trick. People in love hold eye contact for longer than regular friends. Open them up to the idea that there may be something special going on here by holding his gaze and then, when you have to talk to someone else, such as the person behind the bar, hold his gaze for a beat or two longer than normal, giving the impression that you are having to drag your attention away from him to order your drink. This makes you both feel a sense of connection, even though you are the one initiating the contact.

Giving him the eye and getting nowhere?

Basically, unless you have had the secret service tail him for the last six months, there's no way of knowing if he's not responding because he just broke up with someone, is waiting for his girlfriend to arrive or has taken a vow of celibacy; so **don't dwell on any failed flirts.** It's all part of the big whirligig of romantic adventures, so choose to believe something that reflects well on you ('he's overcome by my beauty') rather than the bad stuff ('he thinks I look like a Gorgon'). After all, you'll never really know, so dust off your false eyelashes and try again.

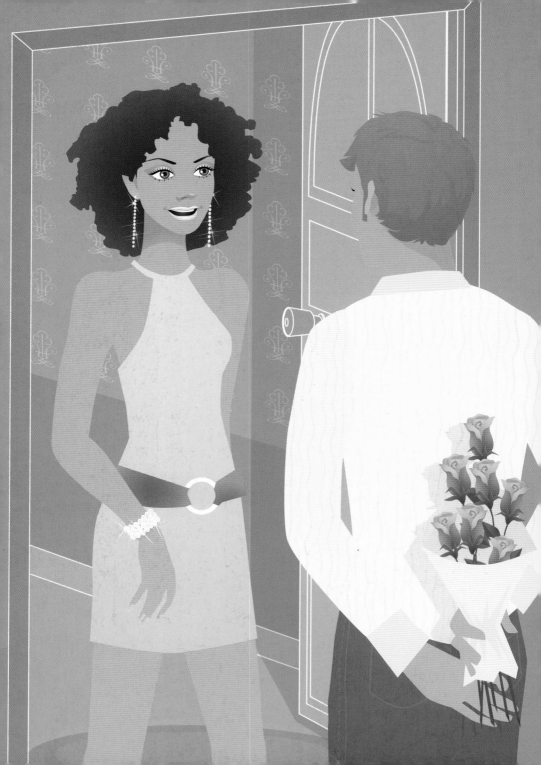

the first date and beyond

◎ Avoid complaining about the weather, the venue, the wine, in fact anything at all. Instead, keep the tone positive and upbeat.

◎ Greet with a kiss on the cheeks. If you start with a handshake you'll never shake off the cold tone of that initial meeting, and anything more is too intimate.

◎ Choose a venue where you can hear each other well and talk easily, such as a quiet restaurant or a walk in the park.

◎ Ask questions, but not just to provide an opportunity to tell your own stories – this will be noticed. Always wait for a complete answer and don't interrupt.

◎ Keep the conversation fairly general at first. Try talking about current events, films or your interests, but avoid too-intimate details, strident views or discussions about money or business.

◎ Maintain good eye contact and avoid looking around the room – it will make you look as if you'd rather be elsewhere.

◎ A sense of mystery will always leave them wanting more. It may be a cliché, but the essential advice is to never reveal too much too soon.

love, life
and knock-back **karma**

When it comes to saying no, do it nicely. The truly charming make everyone feel good, even those with whom they have no interest in developing a relationship. Saying no in a pleasant, clear way is the difference between a brief moment of awkwardness and an agonizing blow to the self-esteem.

Try to follow these simple guidelines:

⭐ Switch on your 'Please leave at the next exit' signal. Cross your arms, move your body away from him, angled toward the door.

⭐ Close down dialogue with brief answers.

⭐ Talk about your boyfriend (real or imaginary).

⭐ Be brief. Say thank you, you are flattered, but politely say that you aren't available. There is never any need to cut someone down in public for the sake of looking clever.

⭐ If you are feeling uncomfortable, trust your instincts. A decent guy will admit defeat and leave after a polite no; someone insistent, despite clear signals, is disrespectful. Don't let them bully you into talking to them. (Enlist the help of a friend, bartender or bouncer if you have to.)

⭐ Finally, take responsibility for your own behaviour and don't use someone as an ego boost. Keeping someone hanging about, accepting a drink from a guy you would never date, giving a smitten colleague the impression something might happen because you're bored at work might not seem so terrible, but put yourself in their size nines for a minute and think it through. If it feels bad to be on the receiving end, you shouldn't be doing it on the giving end. Do you really need the attention that badly? (If so, move to the confidence-building section of this book immediately; do not pass Go!)

the super turn-off!
how to gross-out every guy you meet!

Women are great: we've built empires, raised generations, led armies into battle, floated companies on the stock market and, more often that not, still find a little extra brain space to appreciate a nice-looking pair of shoes. Yet we all seem unable to grasp one of the essential aspects of communication that trips us up in so many of our social dealings, especially with men. We always give TOO MUCH INFORMATION. We seem to imagine that the road to intimacy is paved with bald warts-and-all personal revelations and we are just as likely to subject a man we've only just met to these ear-bending revelations.

Saying you hope one day to live in the country is fine; asking him if he likes 'Ebeneezer' as a boy's name or 'Should twins have names starting with the same letter?' is not so hot. You may think that telling a man your personal problems is **being open and honest,** when in reality it just makes him want to eat his own head so he doesn't have to listen to you any more. He might feel compassion for your grandmother's recent move to an old people's home that she loathes, but men are simple creatures and he may end up wondering whether you are asking him to kidnap her and build her a new house, or if he should be giving you a far-too-intimate shoulder to cry on. The only sure-fire way of having him dive out of the nearest window is to tell that hilarious story of how you used to be totally nuts about some guy and the silly nincompoop got a restraining order out on you but you would never do anything that immature now – not now you have a police record!

Also, for your own sanity, **keep the quizzing to a minimum.** You may feel like a balanced, impenetrable woman of steel when you say, 'So tell me about your last relationship?', but three months later you'll be kept awake at night thinking about that 'amazing' holiday they had

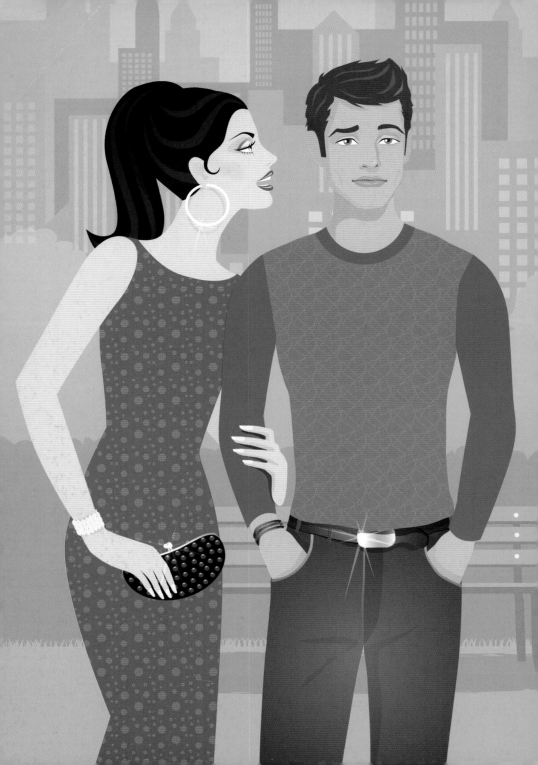

in Morocco and how he thought she was the love of his life until she stole his car. Falling in love makes you vulnerable and you may knit a noose for your own neck. In fact, after a) 'Do you have any sexually transmitted diseases I need to know about?', b) 'Do you have all your own teeth?' and c) 'Can I have some of your chips, please?' what else do you really need to know at this stage? Information on the ex should be delivered as and when it's necessary and even then just enough to understand each other better.

So the basic rule of thumb is: keep a lid on those aspects of your personality better known to you and your friends as **the 'crazies'.** Better to let them out slowly when he is already in love with you.

' Spilling your guts is exactly as charming as it sounds. '

**Fran Leibowitz
(1949–), US journalist**

MEN'S TOP FIVE 'I never want to hear that on a first date'

1. My ex, my ex, my ex, my ex, such a bastard, my ex.
2. Can you pass me that ashtray, please – I need to be sick in it.
3. So when I got over the savage beating my mother gave me, I prosecuted my father for stealing my piggy bank savings...
4. I don't eat meat, dairy, carbs...
5. I need you to donate your kidney to me.

And while we're on men's top fives, here's a few more reasons men decide **not to pick up the phone** to make a date, even if you thought there had been a connection.

1. He was a bit drunk and can't really remember if you are his type. With not enough evidence to support the theory either way, he might just decide to give it a miss.
2. The too-busy syndrome. Men are literal: if they are too busy, they really won't call. And if you have gone on and on about how it's impossible to fit everything into your crazy, busy life, he might think there's no point.
3. He just wanted to see if he could get your number. He had time to kill while he was waiting for his wife's waters to break in the hospital.
4. He can't face the rejection. He just got fired, his dog ran off, he isn't sure how you'll respond, so his ego is taking some time out. The timing was just wrong: if you'd met him on a better week, who knows? Exactly, not you, so forget it!
5. His phone is broken. And if you believe this one, so is your MIND!

If you want to get to a date stage, remember, **men respond well to warmth,** laughing at their jokes (don't we all?), physical encouragement (touching their hands, etc), showing you share an interest – 'A game of tennis sounds fun' rather than screeching, 'Oh God, you love the gym – I totally hate all that narcissistic body beautiful crap!'

But if he doesn't feel moved enough to call, he won't, in which case spend ten minutes sending outraged, vitriolic emails to your mates and then forget about him. As an old Scottish lady of my acquaintance used to say, **'What's for ye won't go past ye.'**

right *place,* right *time*

Of course, there are always the bars and the clubs, but what if you live in a one-horse town and have kissed all the boys already? Obvious answer, try another town. But there are many other ways of bumping into the right biceps.

Think about the kind of man you would like to be with. Is he athletic? Likes animals? Loves to cook? Does he enjoy music, the cinema? Is he creative? Work backward from this point to **the kind of place these guys might hang out.** There may be a local film festival you can go along to (any lectures afterwards are a great way to turn to a bloke and ask, 'What did he just say?'). Do you dream of baking all day and being ravished in haystacks at night? Go to your local farmers' market and see what's on offer.

Wherever possible, give your brain and body a boost, too. Why not try something more unusual, like surfing? It's a fun way to shed pounds and you get to wear rubber! (If you worry about the natural look à la surf, try getting your eyelashes dyed before you go.) The point is, if you frequently bemoan the lack of available men, ask yourself how many of your friends' 'how we met' stories were in bars and how many were down to chance (or dating agencies). Then **throw yourself in the path of fate.**

take an interest
in what he's interested in

So, bingo! You're either past the first meeting and on a date, or you're already drawing his initials on your pencil case. The key to making it stick is to make this person feel good. And a great way to do this is to take an interest in something that he finds truly fascinating, and with most people (especially the male ones), that's himself. Even if you only say, 'A penalty, really? Who would have thought?', he will remember this dialogue as truly fascinating because he was excited and engaged.

Sounds like a tip from *Housewives' Monthly*? The reality is, most men like to feel affirmed and encouraged by a partner (again, don't we all?), so occasionally focusing on something they feel knowledgeable and passionate about sends out subliminal messages of **approval and admiration**. The first thing relationship counsellors tell flagging couples is to get a hobby together; circumnavigate that whole sticky area by cultivating a shared interest before you reach the crisis stage.

he loves sports/motorbikes/knitting and you don't

○ Unless you live in a convent, your beloved won't be the only male in your life; use other men's knowledge to your advantage. Ask them about the offside rule, what match you should really try and see, and what the issue of the day is (usually who's managing whom). They will give you good, informed questions to ask (charm bonus: it will also make these people feel good about you, too).

○ Ask to go along and watch him play in his weekend football game. There's nothing a guy likes more than running about looking manly in front of his girl, and if you make a bit of an effort (even if it's Sunday morning), he gets to show you off to his mates, too. Double score!

○ Train together. If the gym is too much, take up jogging or practising shooting hoops. It's a nonconfrontational, relaxed way to spend time together, which also gives you an endorphin rush, a shared goal, oh, and a chance to show off your bum in shorts.

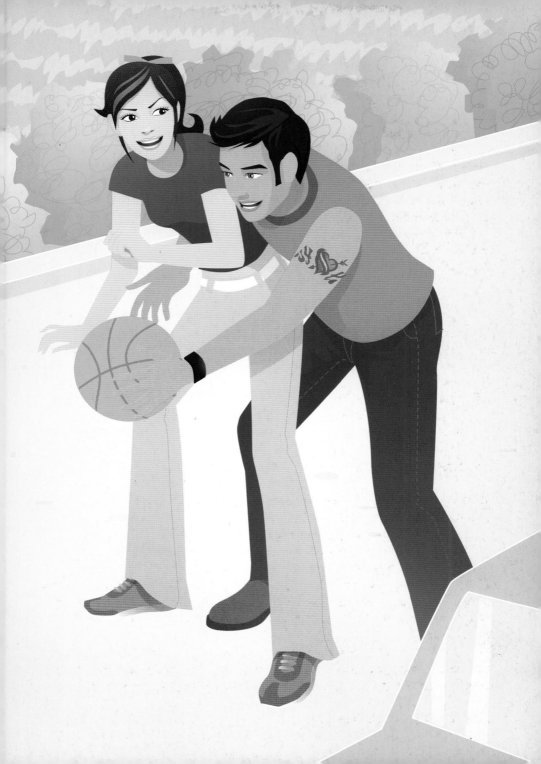

● Draw a line. If he wants to go to the sports bar to watch the match with his mates, or spend a Saturday afternoon watching football in the rain, leave him to it. Don't say, 'Well, what am I going to do?' Sometimes we all need to just be with our own friends, doing our own thing, letting ourselves decompress, and if you are supportive and relaxed about it, he'll look forward to returning to you all the more (especially if you don't call him seven times mid-match to ask him to pick up the dry cleaning on his way back).

● Even if you can't get into the sport, find some common ground. Know enough to understand what it means if his team get relegated or lost a vital match so you can offer tea and sympathy as necessary. Making someone feel understood ('That's a nightmare'), hearing them out ('They sent him off for only breaking a jaw?'), then softly pulling them out of their mood ('I'll fix you something to eat, then let's go out and drink away our sorrows') is a relationship skill worth its weight in gold.

how to make him
fall for you:
the power of *mind-reading*

So you've had a few dates, and you think you might want to take it to the next level, the one that means he introduces you as his girlfriend without going into an anxiety spasm.

To do this he needs to feel that as well as attraction and fun, you have a deeper connection worth exploring. Renowned relationship expert Tracy Cabot devised a strategy for making every man feel like you understand the inside of his brain like a Vulcan mind meld.

follow this technique to make him feel crazy about you:

1 Work out what 'type' he is. Everyone relates to the world through one of these three senses: sound, vision or feelings. Using their way of relating to the world to relate to them will make them feel empathized with and understood.

2 To work out who you are talking to, ask him a few simple questions that will reveal how he filters the world, such as 'How did your drink with your friend Bob go?'.

he may answer along the lines:

VISUAL MAN: 'I've never seen Bob so down. He was all bent over and pissed-off looking. He hates his new boss.'

AUDITORY MAN: 'You should have heard him – he was ranting and raving about this new boss. It gave me a right headache.'

FEELINGS MAN: 'I felt really bad for him – he was really pissed off. He hates his new boss.'

Of course, he may not give such a revealing answer each time, so try different questions that require definite descriptions, such as 'What was your childhood like?' or 'What was your business trip like?'. Just don't do lots at once or he'll think you're undercover for the CIA.

when you know his type, consider:

The **visual man** is interested in, no surprise, what he sees. So use words to reflect this as you talk to him. Tell the visual man you see his point; ask him to look at things from your point of view; when booking a holiday, ask him to picture the two of you sipping a long cold beer as you watch the sun drop behind the mountains. Visual men also respond to pleasant visual stimuli, so try looking groomed and sexy when you go out, buying him a great shirt in a flattering colour, telling him he looks great, or taking him to see a movie when he's had a long day and needs relief.

How you speak to the **auditory man** is as important as what you say. Screeching at the top of your lungs about your day from hell as soon as he walks through the door will set his teeth on edge. Buying him tickets to see his favourite band for his birthday will make him happy. Auditory men are good with language and often have an internal debate with themselves before they compose an answer; try not to jump in with 'Are you listening to me?' while he is doing this, even if you think he's ignoring you. Use phrases relating to sound when you talk to him, such as 'Sounds great', 'I don't like the tone of your voice' or 'I love to listen to you talk about that subject.'

Feelings man finds it easy to express himself emotionally and is often very physically affectionate. He likes sensual pleasures like massage, cooking and exercise, and he might be the only guy who ever responds well to 'How do you feel about us?'. He likes to be touched and to hear you say things like 'I understand how you feel', 'I have a good feeling about us', 'Sorry if you felt I was being cold, I had a bad headache.' Making him feel good with a cuddle in front of a DVD or nurturing him by running a hot bath are all winners.

Finally, you will have a love language, too. There are ways of phrasing you prefer: a visual person doesn't connect as easily when a feelings person says, 'I feel that you aren't paying attention' but they respond better to 'You look like you aren't trying to see my point.' Or if, as a visual person, you dress in your best dress and your sound-driven boyfriend compliments you on your choice of CD instead, **be aware of how you react,** and you might even want to teach him how you like to be spoken to as well. And don't forget that we all have each of these sides, to some degree, as part of our make-up, which is why, when you take that dress off to the sound of that CD, all men will react.

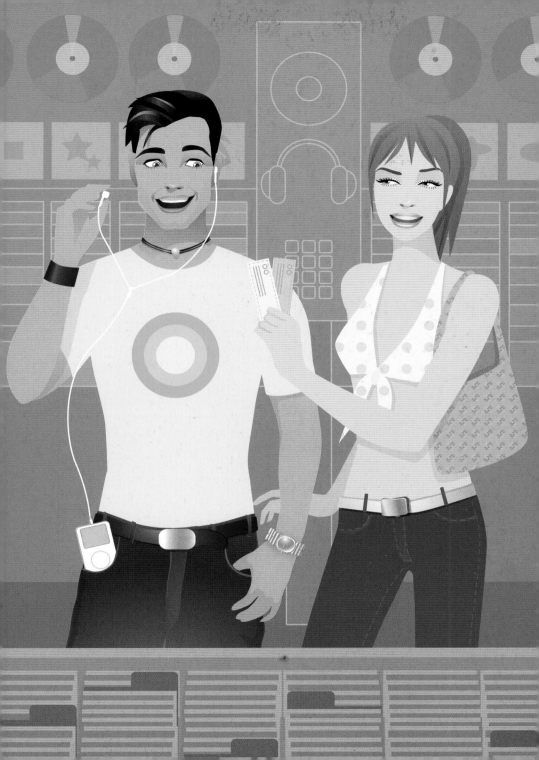

how to keep
the spark alive

Some of us already have the love of a good man. So how do you charm someone who's already seen you in your 'weekend' big pants? Well, having the good sense to occasionally try something unexpected – the old 'keep them guessing' game – helps a lot, so prevent yourself from becoming part of the furniture. And that means you are going to have to carefully plan some spontaneous good times.

First, if you cringe at the thought of trying a new sultry trick on your beloved, consider the fact that flirting makes people feel **attractive and noticed,** and if you never try to recreate that initial buzz, at some stage somebody else will. So think of it as self-preservation.

‘The art of love...
is largely
the art of persistence.’

Albert Ellis
(1913–), US psychologist

dos and don'ts of flirting

Trying to flirt when sports are on TV, you're surrounded by kids or your partner has just had a tooth pulled probably won't work. And doing it in bed may seem like a nice intimate setting but he will just assume that you want sex. Really good flirting is not a verbal way to wrestle them into bed, but a cheeky exchange of fun and attention.

Try flirting when you are out and about together. Put your arms around his waist from behind when you are waiting at the supermarket. Stroke the back of his neck when he is driving. Ask him if he remembers a certain night on a blanket under the stars or tell him you'd love him to wear a specific T-shirt because he looks so darn sexy in it. When you go out for dinner, flash him the strap of a new set of underwear so he can anticipate your return home, giving the evening a sexy edge.

Conversation is essential to charming your partner. It's a common complaint among couples that a person can seem animated and excitable with friends, but **monosyllabic at home.** Make a conscious effort to ask about your partner's day, recall a funny story from your own day (not just a whinge about not being able to find a parking space) and never ever commit the cardinal sin of relationships: cutting them down in public.

Writer Helen Rowland was talking about men when she wrote the following, but it stands for both the sexes, so bear it in mind: 'When a man spends his time giving his wife criticism and advice instead of compliments, he forgets that it was **not his good judgement,** but his charming manners that won her heart.'

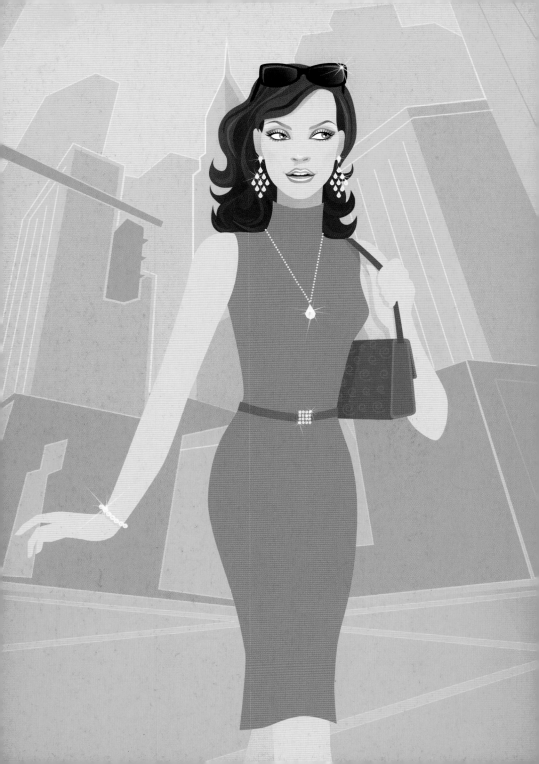

working *your assets* 3

We live in a physical world and to say physical appearance didn't matter in today's society would be an out-and-out lie. But guess what? You decide how attractive you are. Believe it or not, women actually decide how attractive we are to other people by how we are. Research carried out at Brandeis University in Massachusetts, USA, showed that as women age, how friendly and gregarious they were when they were younger influences how physically appealing they become as they get older. Yes, it is a woman's *personality* that affects how attractive people perceive her.

Conversely, the more physically attractive a man is in his youth, the more sociable and amenable people find him as an adult. It seems the way a man looks influences his personality, whereas for a woman the kind of personality she has influences the appearance she develops. That, in itself, has to be a reason to put on a smiley happy face if ever there was one. Still not convinced? Still scowling over your upper thigh measurement? Consider the girl at work or in your group of friends who whines constantly about her big bum/lack of cleavage. Often, these girls have nothing really wrong with the bemoaned part in question – they might even be using it as a way of drawing attention to their tight buns or their pert pair – either way, they become less attractive, and even if they seemed physically modelled on Aphrodite herself when you first met, they have 'talked unattractive'.

‘ When **virtue and modesty** enlighten her charms, the **lustre of a beautiful woman** is brighter than the stars of heaven, and the influence of her power it is **in vain to resist.** ’

Akhenaton
(1352–1336 BC), Egyptian pharaoh

so where do *looks fit in?*

The first thing we do when presented with a new person is to scan them physically. We are already making assumptions about them – and our feelings toward them – before they even say hello. Because she knows she already has her bases covered, the irresistible woman is confident and happy about this fact. And it has nothing to do with having a waist span you can circle with your own hands – it's all about the packaging. So let's start with the easiest bit to change: the stuff you can take off.

dress sense:
why *it matters* what you wear

The ultimate social horror is turning up at a party dressed as a giant egg, only to discover it's not fancy dress. This happens in subtle ways to many people, many times, and they don't even realize. The reason why it is important to adjust your clothing to your surroundings is that you are sending out a message that you understand the social code, and are bright and aware enough to react accordingly.

Attending a job interview at an investment company in a revealing outfit so you can show how sexy and confident you are simply signifies to employers that you are self-obsessed and unaware of proper conduct. The same goes for turning up in a demure suit for a job as a fashion stylist: this quickly communicates you aren't **in tune with your environment.** Only teenagers dress as they like (usually like their friends) and demand to be taken as they are – even at their grandparents' 50th anniversary – and are devastated when no one bats an eyelid. That's because real grown-ups regard it as an endearing phase of childhood.

so what is your wardrobe saying about you?

Outdated clothes that are worn – not '80s retro but '80s without irony or washed to within an inch of their life – communicate that we are either not up to date in our mind-set or can't afford to be. Smelly, tatty or wrinkled clothes say **you lack self-esteem** or are feeling depressed. We've all spent a weekend in ice-cream-stained pyjamas post-dumping, right? This is the same thing on a grander scale.

Super-trendy, barely-off-the-catwalk fashionistas may as well be wearing a sign that says 'Hi, I really care what others think of me and am probably quite insecure'. **Sexy clothes are attention seeking** (duh!), but there is a fine line between 'Check me out' and 'Lock me up!'. Too far on the sexy scale is often a sign of insecurity, as are the comedy ties and Bart Simpson socks that Greg in accounts wears to prove he is **'CRRAAZZEE!!'**.

And at the other extreme, clothes that are totally neutral or boring are saying **'please don't look at me'**.

‘ Put even the plainest woman into a beautiful dress and unconsciously she will try to live up to it. ’

**Lady Duff Gordon
(1863–1935), English fashion designer**

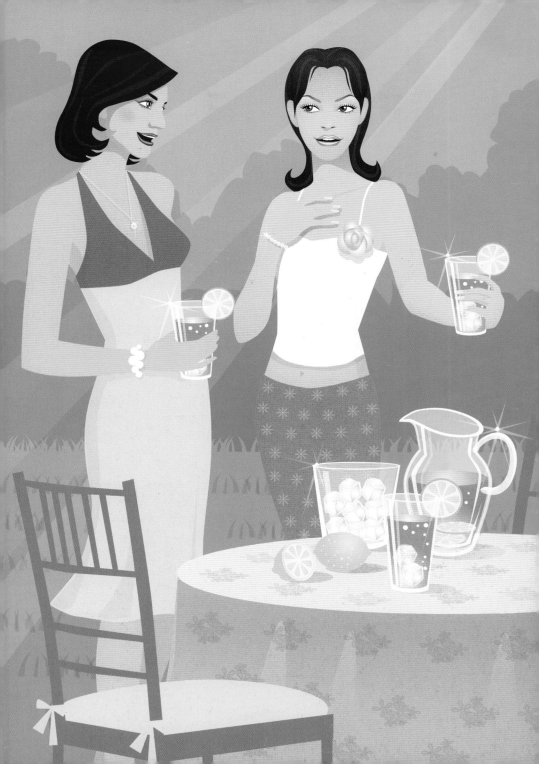

sending out the right wardrobe message

Here are a few simple guidelines for hitting the right fashion note.

1. Consider the event and dress accordingly. For a cocktail party you can dress in your own personal style without offending anyone – well groomed with a sexy backless black dress tells onlookers that you understand the social rules, but are confident enough to show your flair.

2. Make sure everything is clean, pressed and has all its buttons. A safety pin on a broken zipper is fine as an emergency measure, but not as a way of life.

3. Add a dash of colour or a cute accessory (like a vintage brooch) to show confidence, but also to give you something to talk about to handsome strangers or other guests.

4. For sexy dates, wrap the package as you want to be treated. He might not know '70s retro hooker is hot on the Paris catwalk – he may just think you want sex for money and have a nostalgic bent. As a rule, do either legs or décolletage: too much flesh is just cheap and actually detracts from your best feature (whichever you decide that to be). A polo neck with a miniskirt makes long legs a main event, whereas jeans and a blouse showing a little of your cleavage makes it look as though, despite yourself, without even putting all the goods out on the shelves, you can't help but be bloody sexy. You're just that hot.

5. Love that 'lucky sweater' your sister bought you in '84? Yep, it was great. Now it should be kept only for Sunday afternoons in front of the TV and gardening. It won't help you land that job as head of marketing. Zone your wardrobe into winning power outfit, date dynamite and only-on-a-Sunday to prevent you accidentally falling off the taste wagon.

how to *bring* out
your best

You'd be surprised at what grooming can say about you. Unsurprisingly, a lack of hygiene is seen as a sign of depression or self-absorption, showing someone is unwilling or unable to consider how they are perceived by others.

Constantly changing hairstyles and colour is a sign of unhappiness or trying out new identities. Wearing too much make-up (a mask to hide behind) betrays a deep insecurity about yourself. **Tanorexia** (an addiction to fake tan) and an unwillingness to be seen without it, is often a sign of insecurity and inflexibility.

Those who create the best impression use grooming to enhance their greatest features and minimize flaws. They can enjoy experimenting occasionally without playing 'guess who?'. And they don't feel the need to apply a full face of foundation before escaping a burning building. **Appropriate personal grooming immediately signals that you respect and value yourself.**

'Like anyone else, there are days I feel beautiful and days I don't, and when I don't, I do something about it.'

**Cheryl Tiegs
(1947–), US actress and model**

what does **femininity mean to you?**

For some women, it requires a two-hour ritual involving scented gardenia petals and a make-up bag that has to be transported on wheels. For others, it's using a hairbrush once a week. We all have a different set of standards, but usually femininity means that we feel attractive and self-possessed. When we know we look our best, our body language is naturally more open, confident and relaxed, further enhancing the feeling that we are desirable and in charge of ourselves.

The first step towards reaching this happy place is to consider **what kind of woman you are,** and see if that fits in with what you are aiming to achieve.

If you have big boobs and some 'junk in the trunk', there's little point in living off dry crackers and a thimbleful of water in an effort to **get that heroin chic thing** going on. It's the same with having pre-Raphaelite tresses and pale skin – bronzing up and going for a Miami Beach look might not come off as convincing.

It may sound obvious, but work with what you've got. Admit to your friend you think her **double Ds are great,** then buy yourself something floaty and flattering to show off your own pert offerings. So many women spend their lives wishing for something else, only to turn around at 80 and say, 'God, if only I'd realized what a super fox I was! Now I can keep my nipples warm by tucking them into the waistband of my pants.' Whatever you've got, it's temporary, so **make the most of it.**

don't edit
the truth

Gee, us women are great. When we feel low, we look at pictures of 14-year-old models and bemoan our fate. Yet, when we are asked who we think of as being beautiful, we have no hesitation in saying, 'Oh, Isabella Rosellini and Susan Sarandon are goddesses' or 'I loved Andie MacDowell in *Four Weddings*' and 'I think Maggie Gyllenhaal was great in *The Secretary*.' No one ever says, 'That teenager on page seven of *Marie Claire* is fabulous.'

Let's think about it. Most people associate beauties with strength and charisma (the charm of people we've never met). You could point out Isabella's gap-toothed smile, Susan's eligible in some countries for a bus pass, Andie has hair that needs its own trailer and Maggie was probably the class geek. **They all have wobbly bits, and they are all gorgeous.** But they all have make-up artists, and directors of photography lighting them. So stop the pity party and start feeling your own power.

'Beauty comes in all ages, colours, shapes and forms. God never makes junk.'

Kathy Ireland
(1963–), US model

get in the *driving seat*

As any good life coach will tell you, confidence comes from feeling in control of your life, and accepting with good grace the things you can't change. So start your overhaul with a little body workover. Is there anything you can start changing today? Any area that needs a little grooming and fine-tuning? Set aside a Sunday for an overhaul, then vow you will do this maintenance work at least once a month.

While you are overhauling, get yourself down to the make-up counters in your local department store. Ask for a few different opinions and samples while you find a brand with a philosophy and products that are right for you. **We get so used to the same old routine** that it's not until someone asks us whose retro '80s party we went to that we realize we may have let our eye drift off the cosmetic ball. Even from season to season looks change. That foundation we think we need in winter (which would probably be better as a tinted moisturizer anyway) looks patchy and gloopy in summer sun. Also, remember your day and night looks should be as different as, well, day and night. Keep it fresher during the day and add more in the evening: what looks great in a low-lit bar doesn't usually look quite so hot under fluorescent lights of a meeting room.

TIP: have a clear out!

Our skin **changes in tone and texture** as we age, so make sure your foundation is still the right shade and look at your cosmetic colour palette and textures. That shimmery bronzer that looked so high fashion in your early 20s may make you resemble a bowling ball a few years on, and that red lipstick you used in your French existentialist phase when you were a cute freckle-nosed 15? Morticia from *The Addams Family* wants the serial code so she can order in bulk.

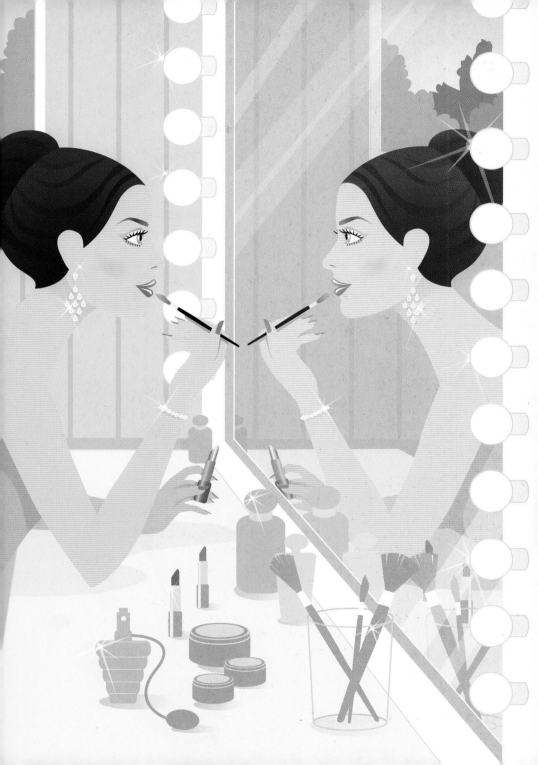

hair, skin, scent
and other beauty boosters

It is a fact that youth is what men find attractive in women, which doesn't mean you have to be young. Emulating the symbols of youth is what counts, as these attributes are read on a subliminal level by the onlooker. Shiny hair, clear skin, bright eyes and teeth, and a waist-to-hip ratio of 0.7 (according to research at the University of Austin, Texas, it's the optimum figure for attracting a guy – high numbers of Miss America pageant winners apparently have this measurement as well) are all desirable. Happily, with modern advances, all your features can be given a helpful boost.

The waist-to-hip ratio is determined by measuring hip circumference at the level of your two hipbones. Divide your waist circumference in inches by your hip circumference in inches. Your waist-to-hip ratio should be below 0.8 for a woman and below 1.0 for a man; however, ratios, like statistics, never tell the whole story.

lustrous locks

Hair is renowned as a **fantastic flirting tool,** whether you have silky waves that you toss knowingly or a buzzcut that shows off the slender, tender part of the back of your neck. And hair that moves and swings will give you natural flirt appeal. Big hair is also very sexy, and a good cut with layers, thick chunks or a long fringe is usually an instant hit with men, assuming it's in great condition, well-styled and clean.

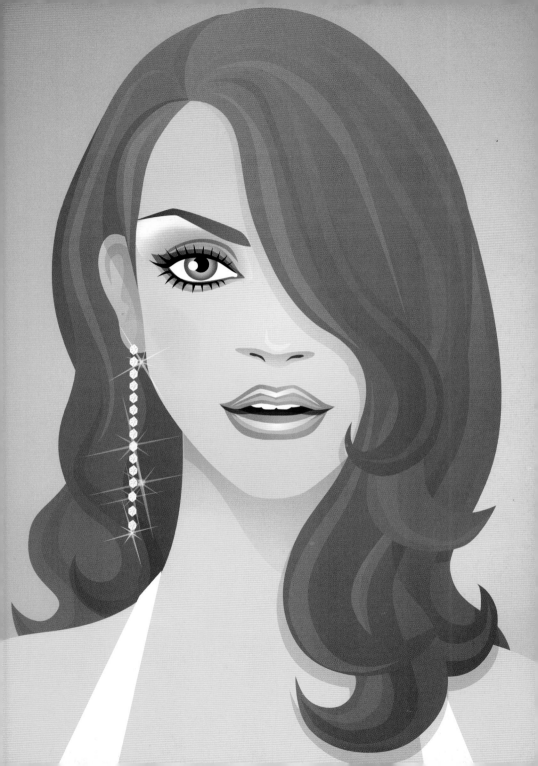

finding the right cut

The key to getting your style right is to **work with what you have.**
Going into the hairdresser's with a photo of some starlet who has a
silky, blunt cut when you have hair that springs out from your skull like
coils will only make them want to stick their scissors in your neck.

How many times have you heard a friend complain, '**It
looked so great when I left the hairdressers!** Now
I look like I'm wearing a Davy Crockett hat.' When that
happens, both hairdresser and client are at fault. The
hairdresser can give a killer blowdry because, as well as
years of training and experience, they are pulling your hair
away from the head with a smoothing tension and not doing
it upside down in a hurry. You should know better than to
pretend you have two hours to spend on your hair every
morning before work. Here are six steps to great-looking hair.

❶ Treat your hairdresser like a therapist. That doesn't mean you
should be sharing your private affairs, but look for one who
you feel understands you, your style and your lifestyle. First, talk
about your hair texture with the stylist. Unless you want to fight
with your hair every day of your life, get a style that works with
the type of hair that you have. If it has a natural wave or curl, is
there a way to create a cut that, on those days when the alarm
didn't go off, a squeeze of product and a scrunch as it air dries
means that it will at least look nice, if not killer?

❷ You also want a look that goes from work to play, day to night.
But you don't need to be a full-on vamp when you're at a sales
conference or at the gym (IBH, inappropriate big hair, is not sexy at
all), but you do want a style that goes from tidy and professional
by day to Wonder Woman sultry by night.

3 Make sure you have the right tools for the job to emulate your new style – your sexy, tousled beach look may be easy as pie to replicate with a decent set of big-barrelled curling tongs. Product is also essential to getting the look right and must match your hair type. Fine hair can't cope with very heavy products – it will end up flatter than when you started – but curly and thick hair will drink it up and be the better for it. Your hairdresser should be able to advise (if not, find a new one).

4 As well as a good cut, consider having highlights or lowlights. Colouring makes thin hair fuller by swelling the hair shaft. It also adds the appearance of depth, texture, richness and a glossy shine.

5 Great condition is essential to your hair's flirt appeal, so once a week do a healing pack of super intensive moisturizer to keep it in tip-top condition and to avoid split ends and brittleness. Even if you are trying to grow your hair, it needs to have 6 mm (¼ inch) chopped off every six weeks to counteract the effects of hair drying and/or straightener abuse.

6 If you have a bad hair day, don't immediately feel defeated; it can often be down to the weather. Humidity causes frizz, dry air makes hair puffy, it often goes flat on a hot day and a lack of moisture in the air causes static. Just have a plan B for these times – a nice headscarf or a sleek, scraped-back ponytail will be a better solution than trying to fight nature and a whole weather front.

bright smile

We've already established the essential nature of a winning smile in almost every social situation. But did you know that white teeth can also add to the illusion of youth? As we age, discolouration from food, drink and habits like smoking dull the teeth. Whitening them is like **turning the clock back.** But make sure your gums are in good shape, too. Young people have bright pink ones so take care of yours – one treatment without the other doesn't have the same effect.

the eyes have it

And of course, don't forget the eyes, those vital flirting tools. Make-up artists agree that the cheapest cosmetic surgery we can all afford is a good pair of tweezers. Plucking your eyebrows opens up the eye and makes it look wider, younger and more appealing. It also means you look **instantly more groomed,** whether you are wearing make-up or not.

soft skin

There's no more obvious sign of ageing than the wrinkling, discolouration and pouching that happens to the skin. The breaking down of collagen, the skin's structural fibre, is a **natural part of ageing,** but what most people don't realize is that exposure to the sun speeds this process up, causing up to a staggering **90 per cent of damage.** It takes ten years for that beach holiday bronzing to show its effects, so you may think you've gotten away with it. Sadly, no. The best thing you can do to give your future self the firmest jawline and unlined eye sockets possible, is to put on a great SPF (a broad spectrum with UVA and UVB cover) every time you leave the house. Treat yourself to a light one designed exclusively for the face so it feels like a treat rather than a chore to use, and then get into the habit of putting it on straight after your moisturizer.

Ageing UVA rays are also transmitted through glass so that warming glow you get from the picture window above your desk is also ruining your face. **Indoors doesn't mean protected.** Face creams loaded with skin-loving, collagen-producing ingredients will also help repair damage you've already done. Look for products containing retinol, antioxidants and vitamin C to give the body's biggest organ (and the one that keeps the other organs in!) the TLC it deserves.

Smooth, hair-free skin is one of the differences between men and women. That's not to say that a full body wax is in order, but something to think about when plotting your beauty maintenance. **As a rule,** only one of you should have a hairy chest.

sleep is your beauty
best friend

Beauty sleep is no myth. Your looks, from bright eyes, clear skin and even thin thighs, are all influenced by the amount of zzzs you catch. A recent study by Columbia University in the USA suggests that the more you sleep, the less likely you are to become obese. People who get less than the recommended amount of eight hours' sleep a night are up to 73 per cent more likely to be obese (although, obviously, your lifestyle counts, too).

Not getting enough sleep will actually **make you eat more,** confounding your dieting plans. If you get only five hours compared to eight, you will have 15 per cent less of the hormone leptin, an appetite suppressant, and 15 per cent more of the hunger increasing hormone ghrelin, making your body scream out for carbohydrates as soon as you wake. Combine this with a hangover and, as alcohol plays havoc with blood-sugar levels, you can understand why you spend the following day craving fried egg sandwiches at 15-minute intervals.

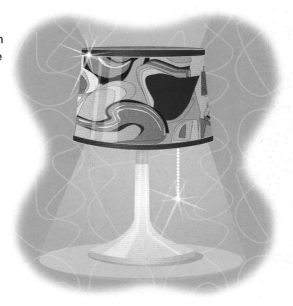

getting a better night's sleep

Think you could be doing better on the sleep front? Even if you get eight hours a night most nights of the week, there might be some things you can do to improve your sleep quality. Consider the following requirements for an ideal rest environment.

keeping it clutter-free

A room that looks like a junk shop will not improve your mood as it will remind you of all you have to do. Make sure you have easily accessible storage – and use it! As well as encouraging you to stay up past your bedtime to send just one last email, computers and TVs in bedrooms disrupt sleep. Red 'standby' lights can also impact on your sleep quality by affecting the brain's ability to switch off. Move the TV out, or at least use black tape to cover standby indicators.

size matters

During the night, we move around up to 60 times while we sleep and your bed needs to give you room to manoeuvre, so buy the largest you can. In addition, most beds only last seven years so don't cling on to it for ever, especially as a tired mattress can give you aches and pains. (If you're looking to buy a new mattress, in general, the higher the spring-count, the better the support.)

soft stuff

Pillows and duvets should be cleaned every four to six months. A mix of duck down for comfort and feathers for support is ideal (although there are great synthetics out there, too). The tog rating on your duvet is a measurement of warmth: the higher the tog, the warmer the duvet. Linen sheets are kindest on the skin as linen is natural and pH neutral. They can absorb up to 20 per cent of their own weight in moisture, thus taking in some of the half pint of water we lose every night in perspiration. With linen and cotton, the higher the thread count, the finer the weave, and the softer it will feel. Anything fewer than 180 thread count will be rough.

atmosphere

The body needs to cool down to allow the core temperature of the internal organs, like the heart and lungs, to slow their rate. That's the reason why hot summer nights can make it so difficult to sleep. The ideal temperature is between 16 and 18°C (60 to 65°F). For the body to activate the 'go to sleep' hormone melatonin, it also needs darkness. Gentle, low lighting in the bedroom, therefore, allows the body to slowly prepare for sleep. Choose low-level lamps that give off a defused light; this also has the advantage of creating a relaxing, intimate mood and, of course, a flattering glow. To wake up with a spring in your step, make sure there is enough light coming into your room to let your body know when to start rousing you from slumber. If it's too dark in the morning you'll have that drugged-up-can't-get-out-of-bed feeling. A special light alarm clock that imitates the onset of dawn can ease you into the day.

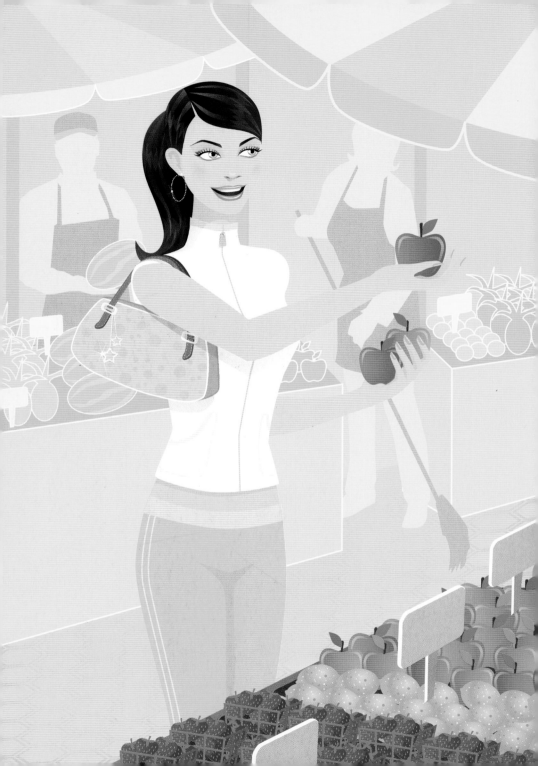

health
and fitness

If you want a guy with a sexy hot bod and six-pack, the fact is, like attracts like. That doesn't mean you have to train for the Olympic swimming team, but in reality if someone is body conscious, they'll be conscious about your body, too. But even if you aren't so concerned about being able to bench press your own body weight, a balanced diet and regular exercise makes everyone, regardless of body shape and weight, more energetic, less stressed, more emotionally stable, have improved skin tone and appear more groomed and polished in their overall appearance. So there's really no excuse for not getting on with it.

nutrition

Basically, what you put into your body is what you eventually get out of it, so giving it rubbish to work with isn't very helpful. Good nutrition is also essential and the best way to maintain a steady weight and stay away from the cookie jar is to **avoid those cravings and panic-eating fits** in the first place. To do this, keep your blood-sugar levels stable. When blood sugar is raised, the pancreas produces insulin to bring it down again (and if this happens too often we can develop diabetes later in life). The short-term effect on our energy is to make us feel **exhausted, irritable and stressed,** and heading back to that cookie jar for a quick hit of energy (and calories).

looking and feeling great

⭐ Water aids digestion, so drink at least 2 litres (4 pints) a day.

⭐ Fresh fruit is the best slow-release energy source. Juiced fruit takes out all the pulp and fibre, which stops you getting a sugar hit from the fructose (nature's naturally occurring sugar).

⭐ Eating protein-rich foods, such as lean meats, cheese, eggs, natural yogurt and fish, for lunch will keep your levels balanced. Refined carbohydrates, like white bread, will cause your sugar level to crash.

⭐ Pulses, beans, lentils, nuts and seeds are all great for slow-release energy. Try them in wholegrain bread.

⭐ Chromium-rich foods, such as shellfish, cheese, baked beans and wholegrain bread, help your body to overcome extreme low blood sugar.

it's the vitamins and minerals that give that shiny glow...
Need more good reasons to eat properly?

VITAMIN B, which is essential for healthy hair, is found in poultry, green leafy vegetables, fish, nuts, seeds, wholegrain products, red meat, potatoes, soya and yeast.

For healthy bones and to avoid osteoporosis later in life, women need to consume adeqate CALCIUM throughout their lives. Unfortunately stress triggers the 'fight or flight' mechanism, switching on the hormone noradrenalin, which in turn causes the body to excrete calcium from the bones, making them weak and brittle. Calcium comes from dairy products, such as milk and cheese. It's also in pulses, canned fish with bones, green leafy vegetables, soya, sesame seeds and tofu. If you use calcium in supplement form, take it with magnesium and vitamin D to aid absorption.

MAGNESIUM is needed for more than 300 biochemical reactions and helps maintain normal muscle and nerve function, keeps the heart rhythm steady, supports a healthy immune system and keeps bones strong. Magnesium also helps regulate blood-sugar levels, promotes normal blood pressure, and is known to be involved in energy metabolism. Find it in apples, nuts, sesame seeds, figs, lemons and green vegetables.

> **VITAMIN C** is an essential antioxidant that repairs the damage of free radicals (molecules in our body that are detrimental to our system) and maintains healthy skin and the operation of many of our main organs. Get it from oranges and other citrus fruit, berries, strawberries, broccoli, cauliflower, raw peppers, kiwi fruit. In fact, all fresh fruit and vegetables contain vitamin C.

If you are too busy to make sure your diet covers all these bases, **take a good all-round multivitamin.** Ensure that the concentration levels are high enough to make a difference (a few cheap brands are so weak they are pointless). Some multivitamins also need to be taken together in order to promote absorption and some should not be taken with food for the same reason. Your **health food store** should be able to advise you.

And, of course, **weight loss** is never far from many people's minds. Assuming you have no special medical problems, such as diabetes, which may need a special approach (talk to your doctor about the safest route for you to take). The US Department of Agriculture (USDA) has reviewed lots of diets and come back to that same old nugget of truth. That you need to **expend more calories than you put in.** Whether you go for a low-fat, low-carb, Glycaemic Index or nuts-and-lemon-juice-only diet, the most effective diets for longterm results have been found to be the ones that limit calorie intakes.

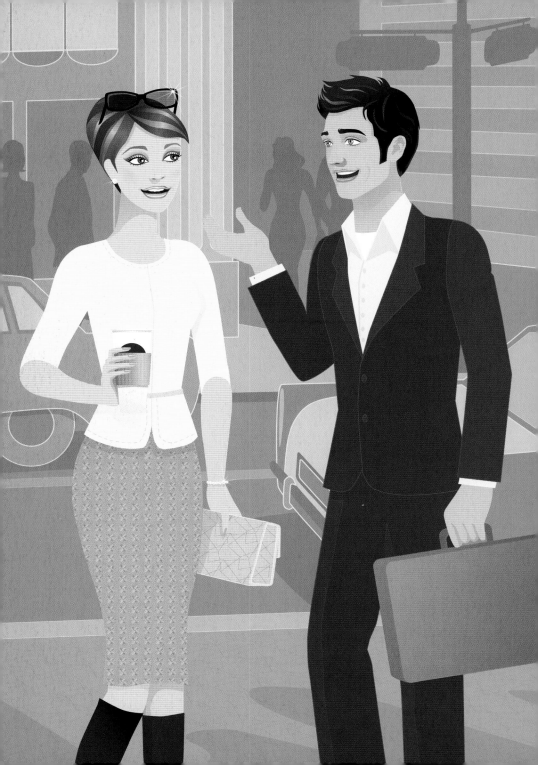

body talk 4

'He who has eyes to see and ears to hear may convince himself that no mortal can keep a secret. If his lips are silent, he chatters with his fingertips.'

Sigmund Freud
(1856–1939), Austrian psychologist

what are you saying, what are they saying?

Before we even open our mouths, we've communicated who we are, what we're looking for and whether or not we think we're going to get it. Like it or not, your body's doing the talking. Non-verbal communication makes up 93 per cent of the messages we send out. Yep, you read that right: only seven per cent of what you say makes up what you communicate.

Do you often wonder why your equally attractive friend is constantly **bombarded by men** in bars, while you're left holding the coats? Or you often find yourself in compromising positions, and not the good kind?

Spend the day looking around you. Are the couple in the restaurant at lunch having a nice meal or arguing about his mother? Is the girl who sold you your paper bored or tired, or eager to serve the handsome guy behind you? Get into the habit of **observing those around you** and trying to read their actions and postures.

It really doesn't matter if your mouth is saying all the right things if your body is screaming the total opposite. Whether you know it or not, people around you are making snap decisions based on your posture and facial expressions. Want to know how to tell your body to shut up? Easy: observe how you are when you are in the company of a close friend. Both of you will be relaxed with open body posture (no crossed arms or hands hovering over the face). You will laugh easily, smile readily and generally seem attentive to them. This is disarming behaviour that makes both of you feel great. Mimic this in times of increased doubt or stress (such as meeting a friend's new boyfriend for the first time) and you will put them quickly at ease and into **'I like you' mode**.

your left ankle told me
you liked me

To be fully effective as an irresistible woman, you need to learn to disconnect what people are saying with their mouths when trying to understand their real desires. People often tell you what they want to hear before you have even said it through their posture, gestures and subtle facial expressions. Most expressions mean more than one thing, and reading posture as well as voice tone will help you draw the correct conclusions.

it's all good...

if the person opposite you is doing any of the following:

PALMS OPEN AND FACING UP – they are relaxed and open to your ideas and are being truthful.

NODDING – they agree, or are simply trying to please you so that you like them.

SMILING – a genuine smile where the cheeks raise, the corners of the eyes wrinkle and the teeth are bared signifies happiness and warmth.

HEAD TILTING – always a good sign, this means someone is interested and listening to you.

LEANING TOWARD YOU – this means someone is interested in you and what you have to say. If they are very interested, their body will lean in and their legs will be drawn back; if someone plonks themselves down in a chair and leans sideways, they are showing that they feel friendly toward you.

WRISTS EXPOSED TOWARD YOU – this action shows vulnerability and can be a very effective seduction tool.

WAVING THEIR ARMS AND HANDS AROUND – this can be good or bad. It means someone feels emotional and passionate about the subject they are discussing. Great, if it's a proclamation of love, but bad if they think it's your turn to pay.

HANDS CLASPED BEHIND THE HEAD – this indicates confidence and a feeling of being comfortable.

GAZE – if they look left, let their eyes sweep over your face and then look to the right, this person is very attracted to you. When they finally hold your gaze and stare for longer than normal you are onto a winner.

CHIN STROKING – someone is trying to concentrate on what you are saying.

BODY FACING YOU – this is a great way to see that someone is focused on you and what you have to tell them, as is them touching you. Things here are going very, very well...

run for the hills...

if the person opposite is displaying these signals:

ARMS CROSSED – this is defensive: they are trying to protect themselves.

HAND ON THE HIP, ELBOW OUTWARD – this is literally creating a physical barrier saying 'stay away'.

FROWNING – can be a sign of anxiety, anger or dislike.

HIDDEN HANDS – hiding your hands is a sign you are holding back or keeping something secret.

RUBBING THEIR NECK – someone is lying or storing repressed thoughts.

TOUCHING/RUBBING THEIR FACE – this may mean someone is not telling the truth and is feeling uncomfortable. If they cover their mouths or eyes during or after speaking, they are trying to break contact after a lie. And if they are rubbing their eyes, they have had enough of what you are saying and want you to stop.

FEET OR LEGS POINTING TOWARD THE DOOR – they are thinking 'Get me out of here'.

SHOULDER SHRUGGING – this usually means someone is indifferent, lying or not being straight with you. However, raising – but not dropping – your shoulders is submissive, and means 'I'm harmless'.

HEAD JERKING – while they are talking, this means they are uncomfortable with what you are saying and are literally trying to pull their head away.

HEAD SCRATCHING – the person is unsure about their thoughts, the question you asked or how to respond. Try asking in a different way.

KNUCKLES CLENCHED – this is a clear sign of anger. If the clenched hands hide the thumb, they may be feeling worried, threatened or intimidated.

ROCKING BACK AND FORTH – this is a display of discomfort, showing anxiety or impatience. It's a self-soothing technique designed to make a person feel better.

OUTSTRETCHED LEGS – this person wants to dominate and be the centre of attention.

NOT MEETING YOUR GAZE – the more we like someone, the more we look at them. The reverse is also true. If they meet your gaze but with a squinty, hard look, they may be angry with you.

LEANING AWAY OR STEPPING BACK – they aren't interested in you and are letting you know it by literally pulling away. Standing far away may show that they are feeling threatened.

IN YOUR BODY SPACE – unless you have invited someone into your space (which means you are probably by now sucking face), a person who gets too close may be self-absorbed or narcissistic and uninterested in how you feel, or intentionally trying to intimidate you. Back away fast!

FIDGETING OR TAPPING FEET – can mean anxiety or impatience, but always means someone is uncomfortable in some way.

TOUCHES YOU TOO HARD – angry or competitive people do this; avoid them.

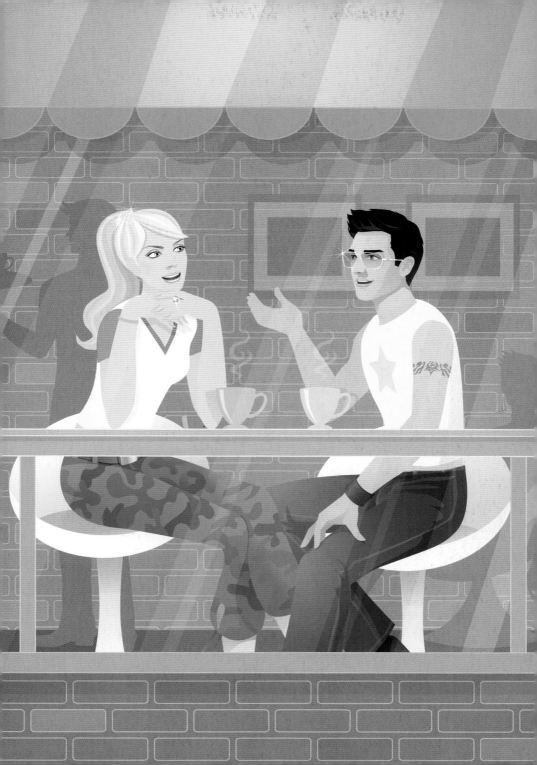

mirroring

Now you know how to read other people's body language, here's how to use your own to great effect. As far as techniques go, this is the master in making people feel good about themselves and, more importantly, you. When people are in love, they often do this naturally by working on a task in harmony (like washing the car or cooking), finishing each other's sentences or planning trips.

This harmony usually occurs because both partners feel **understood and appreciated.** And you can use this natural occurrence to your own advantage by mimicking it when you meet someone. If someone crosses their legs, subtly cross yours; if they lean their chin on their hands, ditto. You might think it looks really obvious but as long as you don't turn it into a game of **'Simon Says',** it will subliminally make them feel that you are in tune. Repeating phrases they use, or acknowledging their feelings, 'I can see why you would be frustrated with your boss', all make them feel comfortable and connected to you.

homework

Find you forget all this stuff in the heat of the moment? Try this: rent a movie you've never seen (best if it's one with a lot of dialogue – it's easy to cheat by imagining what people are feeling if they have just had their car blown up or been stranded on a desert island), and watch it through **with the sound down.** Try and work out what is going on by studying their facial expressions and body movements (not plot points such as 'Peter has fallen into the well', but are they angry, suspicious, loving or hiding something?). Watch again to see if you missed anything, then turn up the sound. Practising will hone your skills and build your confidence in your body-reading abilities.

look me in the eye
and tell me I'm not a Goddess

Using eye contact to send very clear messages is the key to ultimate success when trying to win someone over. Avoiding it can make you seem shifty, deceitful and uninterested, none of which should ever be a part of the irresistible woman's repertoire. If you find eye contact hard to maintain or initiate, remember that run-in you had (and everyone has them occasionally) with a man or woman who did the too-important-to-be-talking-to-you routine. They are always looking away – over your shoulder, at their phone or scanning the room – and regardless of how interested they say they are, you feel furious and unappreciated by the time you part.

Think of a time when you thought someone was lying to you (or even, when you know you were lying to them). Usually the fibber will cast their eyes up, down, to the side – basically anywhere other than at your face. Practise **holding their gaze,** or staring more intently at people you already know, and see the effect that has. They may relax and become warmer with you, and leave feeling more 'understood' or considered by you. And finally, **don't go overboard:** an unbroken stare can be like a car hurtling toward you with its headlights on full beam – it makes people want to cover their eyes and take cover.

‘As the tongue speaketh to the ear, so the gesture speaketh to the eye.’

From *The Advancement of Learning*
by Francis Bacon
(1561–1626), English philosopher and essayist

touch

– it's not all about sex

The power of touch can be harnessed in all your relationships, not just the ones that you might expect to be physical. There is a fine line, however, between appearing warm and seeming needy, or like the office pervert.

Touching must be respectful and appropriate – never try to touch someone who clearly doesn't like it. If you are unsure, they will soon let you know; some people are aching for a friendly pat on the arm and are just too shy to initiate it, while others would rather walk through life in a nineteenth-century diving suit and find your charm offensive, confounding your intentions. So try it once and **see the reaction you get.**

A light touch or squeeze on the back, arm, hand or shoulder all communicate warmth and consideration. You obviously need to moderate your gestures to the person – slapping your boss on the back after a presentation could quite easily have you cleaning out the stationary closet over the weekend. You can also use touch to **emphasize a point,** such as squeezing a friend's hand when you tell her that you are truly sorry you spilt red wine on her white dress, but don't use it to get attention, especially when that person is already talking to someone else – they will end up feeling like the rope in a tug of war.

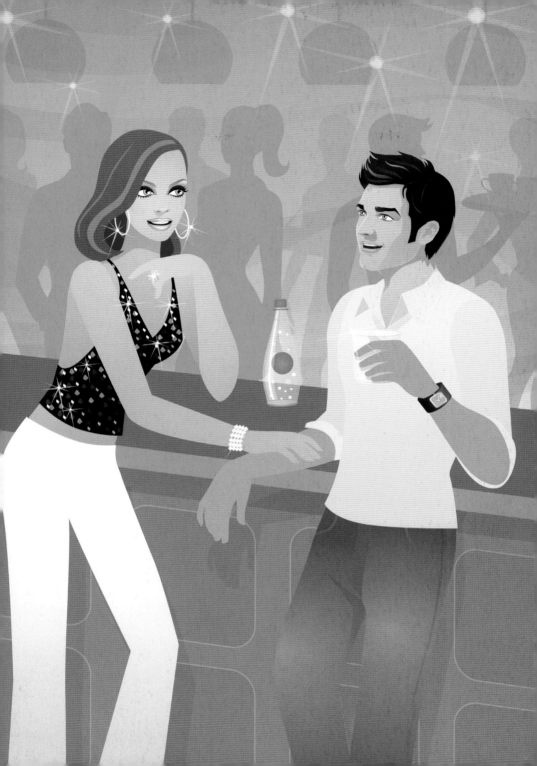

you are now
irresistible...

So now you can read people, here's how to make them drift like iron filings to a magnet.

There are ways in which your body language **subliminally affects other people,** by making them feel you are welcoming, interesting and someone they need to know.

Keep your hands open and exposed, ensuring that you are displaying none of the 'Run for the Hills' postures mentioned on page 74. Every now and then **take a mental audit** of your posture and see if nerves or uncertainty are causing you to use any of these postures (such as the classic folded arms). If it's your default position at a party and you find it nigh on impossible to break, try holding a glass of wine to at least open your body up a little. Don't stand in corners or hide behind people, and if you want someone to come over, don't forget to tractor-beam them with a look and warm smile.

' Charm is the quality **in others** that **makes us** more **satisfied** with **ourselves. '**

Henri-Frédéric Amiel
(1821–1881), Swiss philosopher

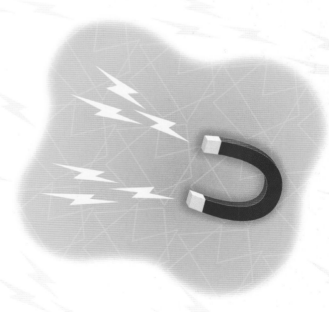

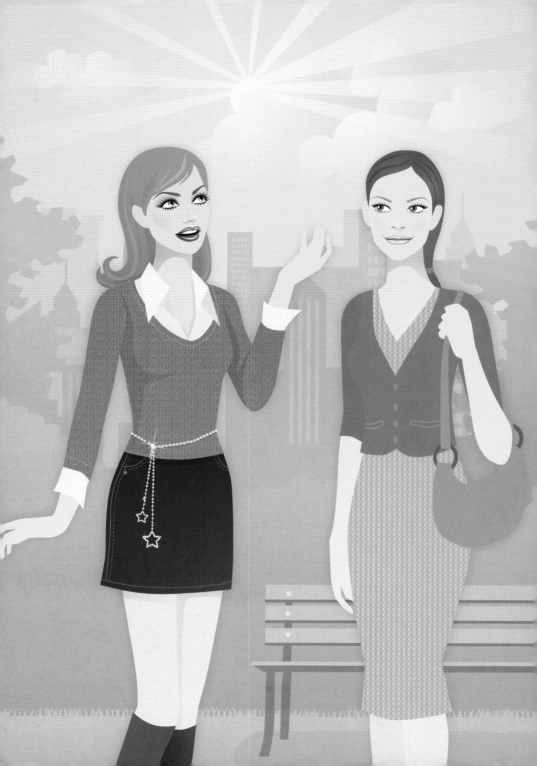

communication *skills* 5

> **' Don't knock the weather: Nine-tenths of people couldn't start a conversation if it didn't change once in a while. '**
>
> **Kin Hubbard (1868–1930), US cartoonist, humorist and journalist**

what you say counts

Even the most beautifully groomed, stylish and chic among us must open our mouths and speak at some point. After the initial hit of appearance, this is the time when we start to make our lasting judgements about others; and, frighteningly, when a stunning vision of sexiness can become a vapid bore or fascinatingly, an Average Joe becomes a must-have mate.

The great thing about verbal communication is that it gives you a chance to engage your brain and reveal your personality, allowing you the chance to raise your stock value, whatever nature gave you to work with. But even more than what you say, *how* you say it influences people's final decision about who you are. When they talk, people tell us things, and the stuff we should really be listening to isn't usually their words. Spoken words makes up only seven per cent of our message with a staggering 38 per cent of our communication skills made up of 'paralanguage', meaning the intonation, sighs and body language that are part of our speech.

Lillian Glass, PhD, is a psychologist and expert in the field of communications, and she believes there are **four key ways** in which people tell us who they really are. The first is the **speaking code**, which is what they say; the second is the **vocal code**, which is how they sound when they say it, such as the pitch and tone of their voice. The other two are **facial expressions** and the **body language code** (see chapter four, pages 70–81 for more on these). Regardless of what a person is saying in words, Glass says there is always some 'emotional leakage' through their voice, posture and facial expressions. The irresistible woman should learn to read these codes so she knows if her potential boss/date/friend will actually call when they said they would.

how to crack the *speaking* code

Ever wondered why you left a discussion with someone, running their words over and over in your mind but feeling unable to pinpoint why they left you uncomfortable or irritated? It may be that they were sending out a subliminal or contradictory message so you got their meaning all right, but can't pin it on them. Learn to recognize some of these sneaky types and trust your instincts when you meet them.

'what a lovely girl you are'

Unless this person is 105 and can't be bothered to keep up with modern vernacular, they are trying to show they disrespect you. They may be a misogynist and think women should only be used for breeding, or perhaps they are just plain stubborn. Don't let them goad you; this is about them, not you. Avoid them if you can. If not, report them to human resources or gently ask them if they have bought any gramophone records from the hit parade recently. Sometimes **a little good-humoured teasing can show them how ridiculous they sound.**

'I disagree'

What, to everything? To the suggestion we should get some coffee? A contradictor is competitive, playing power games, or trying to let you know they don't like you. If you find yourself doing this to a partner or friend, **have a little friendly chat with yourself and find out what you are really angry about** because, in the long run, this type of behaviour always makes the contradictor seem smaller than the butt of their hostility. Another version of this person is the one who insists on peeing on your bonfire. If you say, 'I'm going on holiday to New York for a week – I'm so thrilled!', they say, 'Oh, what a shame, anyone who travels a lot could have told you, you'll just get over the jet lag and have to come back. Never mind.' Plot their death in your mind, but give them a pat on the arm and say, 'Oh you're so sweet to care! But I'll just get round that by staying up all night.' Covering them in honey will ground them, and stop them from buzzing up into your ear and stinging you again.

'I was only kidding!'

No you weren't! if someone tells you that you look so much better with a little padding, they generally use this ploy to make you seem uppity and touchy. Don't let them affect your sense of self and resist the urge to say, 'So do you'. Instead, pat your tummy and say, 'Aren't I lucky?'. The **person who does this is either feeling jealous and resentful** or trying to communicate something to you that they are too afraid to say honestly, because they either know it's mean **or they are frightened of your reaction.** Consider if the hidden message behind their words has any validity, or ask yourself if it is their rapid weight gain that is causing them to look at you with jealous eyes. **(You look great by the way.)**

'and then she said...'

A little bit of gossip is good for the soul, as it binds social alliances and creates confidences. But that tends to be harmless 'Oh, Jill had her baby' rather than 'Oh, Jill had her baby and strangely he looks nothing like her husband but bears an odd resemblance to Phil in Bought Ledger.' A gossip can focus on you and smother you with attention, and before you know it she'll have your medical records in her bag, swearing secrecy, before lurking by the photocopier waiting for someone to whisper about your 'rash'. **This is usually a sign of envy, competitiveness and jealousy.** The best way to handle these people is to stay neutral and ask them a personal question. They will soon give you up as a lost cause.

'and then I said...'

They love the sound of their own voice and they think that you love it, too. **No detail of their sandwich is too minute to extrapolate upon.** These types should hang out with the people who say nothing and give away no personal details as they are essentially about the same thing: themselves. Both types of people are insecure and self-obsessed, demanding a lot of attention through the persistent flow of information, or lack of it.

Make sure that you aren't guilty of any of these unpleasant techniques; they are in no way the territory of the charming, but being able to recognize the motivation of the woman who makes you uneasy at work, or the doctor who makes you feel about five when you ask him for a repeat prescription for your contraception, will help you rise above their behaviour and not let your irresistible crown slip. This is not about giving in to their tactics; **it's about being able to spot a toxic talker at 50 paces and start walking in the other direction.** The best way to be charming is to surround yourself with people you want to be nice to.

reading it wrong

We've all been duped. We've all gone out with a guy thinking he has a beautiful soul when really he turns out to be a selfish coward. But rather than berate ourselves for missing the signs, staying in every weekend going over the hideous details ('How could I have believed those marks on his neck were a scarf burn?'), we should chalk it up to experience and be out there tuning up our antenna.

And remember, unless we are trained clinical psychologists, **being able to see through someone who has decided intentionally to deceive us is quite unlikely;** accusations with no good reason gets us the nickname 'paranoid'. Plus, our biology can fox us; if you fall for a wide-eyed, boyish charmer only to realize you are one of a harem, **remember we are programmed to see 'baby' faces as innocent.** How do you think Leonardo diCaprio gets away with such ladykiller antics?

homework

It has been proven that you can improve **your people-reading skills and therefore become a more accurate judge of character** by getting out there and spending time with people. Someone accustomed to social interaction will be better placed to read them, so just trying to work out if the pizza guy fancies you 'cos he delivered your pizza five Friday nights in a row and said your pyjamas were nice isn't going to give you the power of emotional ESP. Get out with a friend, meet some people and then compare notes on what you think they are like to see how good you're getting at developing these skills.

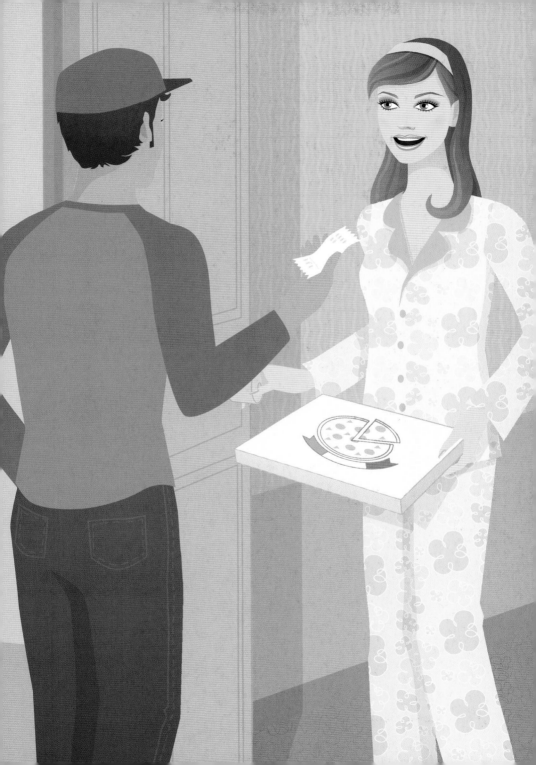

don't you use that tone of voice with me, young lady...

We've all been on the end of that one, and usually with some justification. When your dad wouldn't let you go to the rollerdisco unless he dropped you off outside the door, you probably let him know you were less than enthusiastic about him ruining your chances of kissing the captain of the football team by destroying all your credibility. And when we agree to spend the weekend painting our grandparents' spare bedroom, our tone of voice – no matter how falsely chipper – probably lets them know we'd rather be having a lie-in.

When meeting someone for the first time, think about these voice qualities:

- Is the pitch of their voice high or low?

- Are they loud or does their voice fade out in a softly spoken manner at the end of the sentence?

- Choose a word to describe the quality, such as harsh, gravely, nasal, whiny, tremulous.

- What style do they employ? Is it flirtatious, sugary, slow with pauses or monotone?

Once you start thinking about a person's voice, **it soon becomes obvious how much you can understand about their state of mind and attitude.** Here are a few things to consider once you have categorized your answers.

PITCH: A high-pitched voice isn't a good quality in a man or woman and usually signifies immaturity, aggression, insecurity or weakness (although body-code expert Lillian Glass also points out that it can be linked to arrested development relating to a childhood trauma, so don't rest all your judgements on this one quality).

Low-pitched voices in both sexes are seen as sexier, more capable. But artificially dropping the level of the voice can seem strained and make you sound as if you are standing in a hole.

VOLUME: Voices that start off audibly but tail off later on show that the person has a lack of conviction that what they are saying may be of interest and they are usually suffering from low self-esteem. This can often happen to someone who has just decided to speak up in the team meeting for the first time, but halfway through suddenly wonders if they should even have opened their mouth.

Loud people can be insecure, demanding attention and making their presence felt. Or they may just have been one of a very large family and are still in the habit of having to squawk, 'Hey, that's my piece of toast!'. Conversely, **a quiet person may be frightened of drawing attention to themselves, have no confidence in their ideas or be communicating an inner sadness.**

But here is the catch: both quiet and loud categories can also illustrate an incredibly manipulative and angry person. A softly spoken person insists that others lean in and focus on them just to hear them, which is as intentionally controlling as the bully who barks orders or talks over those around them.

Style is also a good indicator of character or state of mind. It's not hard to work out that a shaky, tremulous voice is a sign of upset; someone whose voice always goes up higher at the end of a sentence, making everything they say sound like a question rather than a statement, is uncertain of themselves while someone who talks quickly may be anxious, and a lack of confidence makes them want to finish their statement quickly in case you lose interest.

Attacking voices, which loudly burst forth with judgements, gravely or relentless, manic voices usually belong to angry and bullying people, who are selfish and self-absorbed. If by chance, they are remotely aware of those around them, **they are often competitive and are trying to undermine and unnerve others.**

Breathy, sexy voices are usually put on to manipulate the listener, but if this person is using them on you, they'll use it elsewhere, so don't be seduced – **unless it's genuinely intimate, then be as seduced as you like.**

This is similar in effect to that of **the sugary baby voice; these people are essentially making themselves seem vulnerable** to appeal to your instincts to take care of them. But don't: they are not to be trusted and are often angry and hostile people.

Depressed or sad people often have a voice that is flat and monotone, but this can also show that a person is not really interested in those around them and is arrogant and aloof.

A clipped, sharp way of speaking can be the sign of someone who feels superior to you, believing there is nothing to learn from you, showing them as buttoned-up and repressed.

Assuming it is not a regional accent, **a very slow speaker may be trying to hold the focus on themselves** and control the flow and pace of the conversation.

Most people's voices change with the situation to some degree. For example, after a hectic day alone with the kids, a care-giving parent might 'babble' and offload stories of spilt juice and fist fights in the playground without so much as a 'How was your day?'. That very same parent may be a loving, thoughtful listener, given a day off and a chance to unwind, so as well as using these vocal codes to decode strangers, use them to work out what mindset those you know are in and if they need help or support. You'll seem like the ultimate irresistible mind-reader if, unbidden, you give encouragement and affirmation to a friend whose statements lately all seem like questions, or offer to babysit for a flat-toned, worn-out parent.

It's also worth considering why **most people's voices change and develop as they do.** The shy stutterer at school, for example, may impress you with deep sonorous tones ten years later at the school reunion, after they found a rewarding career or a sport that helped them gain confidence. Think back over your own verbal experiences, such as sullen teenage mumbling, and use them as a guide for areas in your life that you could try to improve upon. Make sure you are aware of how your voice often reveals more than your words: **listen to yourself.**

how to be pitch perfect

A winning tone of voice in men and women is of a rich, low pitch with an enthusiastic bounce to it, expressing a full range of emotions. **It is strong, doesn't falter and shows confidence, at the same time making us confident in them.**

When you know who you are and like yourself, you don't have to hide, sell or exaggerate anything. The first step to talking like a winner is acting like one; so if you find yourself stumbling over excuses of how the dog ate that report to your boss, you really have only yourself to blame. **The best way to make your words sound good is to be as good as your word.** Make your promises count, admit to mistakes without attempting to palm off blame and keep your commitments. This immediately makes your words meaningful. When you choose to pay a compliment, make it genuine and specific. Ask lots of questions and don't assume you know the answers. Be clear about what you want. Remember that being a good communicator is often more about being a great listener.

all the
good stuff

So now you understand what people say and how they say it, it's time to look at the conversational techniques that make you the most interesting and desirable of guests. The key here is often not what you put into your dialogue, but mainly what you leave out. In the case of charming conversation, the thing to always remember is that people love to talk about themselves; they feel confident about knowing their subject well, have a profound interest in the theme and even if they only catch your name, make them imagine that you are the most fascinating person they have met in an aeon.

But don't overdo it! It's essential that you offer up some personal information and opinions or **you will seem more sycophant than suave.** But it is the way that you direct this flow of information that makes all the difference.

So let's start with **the ladies' favourite: the compliment.**

everything is relative

When it comes to charm *always* be relevant. 'Relevant' should be your magic charm word from now on if you truly want to become irresistible. Make sure whatever you say has some resonance with your audience. Compliments are essential for letting someone know that you have noticed them, are interested in them and are focused on their needs. But a bland compliment can make you seem utterly insincere, as overusing the same phrases dilutes their intent. For example, when you ask your boss what they thought of your report and they say 'Great', you can feel a little disappointed. If they had said, 'Very thorough, I was impressed at how well researched your statistics were', you'd feel like they have paid close attention and valued your efforts.

So practise sharpening up your technique:

BLAND: 'Your hair looks nice.'
BOWLED OVER: 'Those blonde lights really make your eyes look blue.'

BLAND: 'I liked your speech.'
BOWLED OVER: 'Your take on quantum physics was really fascinating; I was captivated!'

BLAND: 'Nice dress.'
BOWLED OVER: 'What a stunning dress, you have such a great eye for choosing vintage pieces.'

Try using this technique **when you say thank you,** too; **make it a relevant thank you,** to make it really count. Say, 'Thank you for a delicious dinner, it was such a treat to have a home cooked meal.' Or 'Thank you for taking the time to go over this work with me, it really helps me understand it better.' Instead of a social nicety, **your 'thank yous' will have real resonance and leave the other person with a warm glow.**

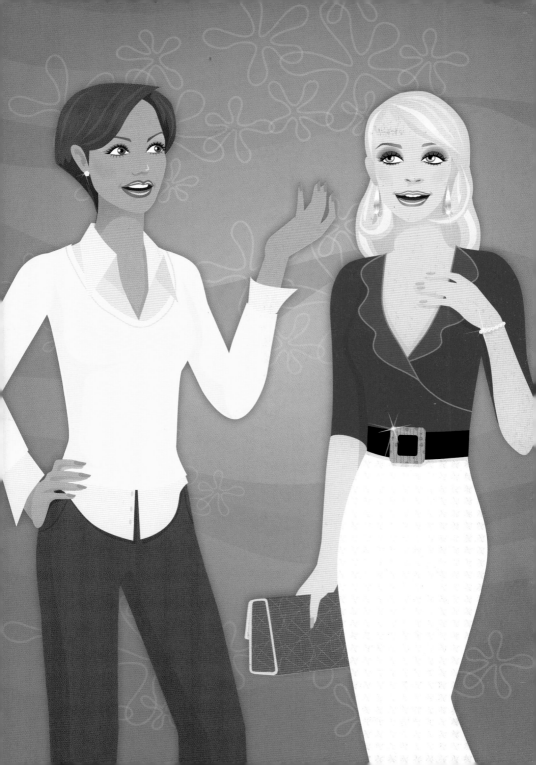

expect *the best*

Most people are more than aware of their own shortcomings. If you are in a position of superiority, be encouraging, not critical. For example, if you are teaching a new skill, say 'Good try, you're getting there. Now take another look at this area' rather than 'Oh no, that's all wrong; you have got a lot to learn.'

If you need to deliver some criticism **make sure you start positively, and be helpful,** such as 'You are really mastering the order process. I find it also helps to make duplicate copies for my own file, that way you can always keep track.' **Everyone had a teacher whose lesson they raced to because they made them feel good,** even if they weren't top of the class. And lots of peopled dropped a beloved subject because they felt defeated.

' I've learned that people will forget what you said, people will forget what you did, but people will never forget how you made them feel.'

Maya Angelou
(1928–), US author and poet

 98 *communication skills*

I feel good, you feel good

A common mistake, but one we all make, is to assume that if we feel good, so too does the other person. Everyone has been on a date where the other person has indulged in a monologue about their love of football, or has a friend who talks about the intricacies of their surgery, oblivious to the fact that you have been wriggling around in your seat with boredom or nausea.

They leave feeling heard, understood and possibly a bit lighter from dumping their emotional load. Asked about the few hours they just spent, they might say it was great while you are hastily deleting their number from your phone. Draw on this experience to **remember that conversations should be two-way** and **MUTUALLY** interesting; be aware of the other person's enjoyment level, even if they are smiling away cheerily. They might just be too polite, or too shy to openly weep with exhaustion in front of you.

The truly charming person is always aware of how other people feel and acts accordingly. Finding themselves in a conversation about tennis in front of someone with no knowledge or interest in it, they ask that person about their favourite pastime, making them feel included and considered. Think of it as passing a hot potato on a cold day; **make sure everyone gets that nice warm glow in turn,** so they all leave feeling good about themselves, and of course, you.

just can't **help it**

Sometimes, when we are under pressure or a situation means a lot to us, we can confound all our good intentions. In an interview for a job we want, meeting a partner's parents or with a recruitment agent you hope can change your career, we exhibit behaviours such as scratching our nose, looking away, rubbing our neck – any basic kind of fidget.

They can interpret this nervousness as being shifty, even if you are speaking straight from the heart with the best of intentions. **The key here is to 'know thine enemy'; basically, you.** You need to make an exerted effort to curb this twitching. Try this exercise to work out what you need to say, so you can leave a little brain space for controlling those urges.

homework

Sit with a friend and ask them to run through the meeting as if they are the interviewer/ doctor/potential mother-in-law. **Refine your answers so you waffle out your first lot of nervous replies, making a note of when you have said something pertinent and to the point.** Try this a few times until you feel confident that you are 'on message'. Although you can't predict all the questions, you will feel more prepared, allowing you to be more confident and able to concentrate a little on stopping that 'scratch'.

making someone
feel smart

When you like someone and hope they will like you too, make sure you feed them lots of 'hooks'. When asked about your job, don't just answer 'marketing'. Instead, expand, either with the location of your offices ('Right downtown, great for pay-day shopping'), what it involves ('We're working on a big campaign for a car company right now – I'm learning more than I ever thought about four-wheel drives'), or how you got there ('I did a law degree at City College but I love the social aspect of what I do now').

All of those answers have facts littered through them that the other person can expand upon. This will put them at ease and **help them feel like they are asking great questions.**

The ideal way to make them feel supersmart is to get them onto a subject they know a lot about; **namely, anything to do with themselves or their own experience.** When a chance presents itself, ask their opinion, or simply switch the dialogue in their favour. On their own turf, they are more likely to flourish.

'We like so much to hear people talk of us and our motives, that **we are charmed** even when they abuse us.'**

Marie de Sevigne
(1626–1696), French novelist

making someone
feel extra-special

Research shows that using someone's name throughout your conversation makes that person feel appreciated and special. In a group situation especially it helps create a link between you and that person, making you stand out from the rest. (Of course, don't use it in every sentence – that might just make you sound a bit odd.) This also helps you remember their name, so you won't find yourself blankly staring at them, while you scan through your mental address book next time you meet.

Once you have mastered this technique, try adding in a few personal references, **letting them know they are special enough to have retained some information about them.** Ask them about their dog, the vacation they were about to take last time you met, or their kids. You may think you can't store this kind of information about everyone you meet, but you will be surprised how much you have retained when you apply yourself. Just **one focused, detailed question will mark you out as a considerate and thoughtful listener** and leave them with a warm feeling.

TIP: got a terrible memory?

Next time you are at a conference or work soirée, make sure you collect business cards. When you get home, take five minutes to jot down a few personal details such as their home town, spouse's name or any acquaintances you have in common. Next time you expect to see them, you can **jog your memory with your own little flash cards.**

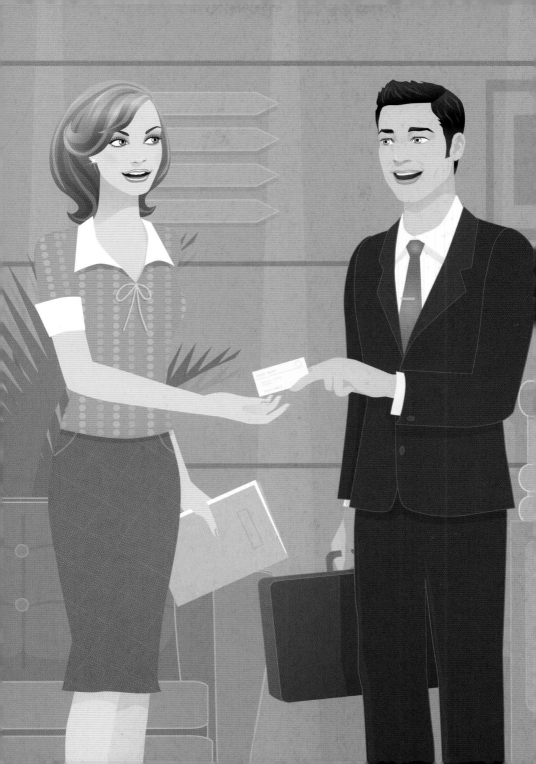

communication
mishaps

Sometimes our intentions start out well and then we just slipslide into a little bad behaviour. Oops! Perhaps your sister just knows exactly which soft spot to press and before you know it, you're going for the jugular. Think about the subtle ways that you may have let yourself down and eradicate them from your repertoire.

never respond to the backhanded compliment

This is the territory of the truly weak. Knowing that the situation calls for a few words of praise, the master of the backhanded compliment says things like 'Wow, what a beautiful wedding dress, and to think we thought you'd never get into it!' or 'I think the cake you made looks lovely under the circumstances.' Handle these nasty barbs by **only ever responding to the good bits with a warm thank you;** the rest is designed to make you respond (and look like you are overreacting) and upset you. If you do so, they've won. Think of it as a sugar-coated cyanide pill. Suck off the sugar and spit out the rest. **(IT'S GUARANTEED TO INFURIATE THEM.)**

never dwell on the bad stuff

No matter how tempting it would be to elaborate gleefully, when someone brings it up at after-work drinks, that the office bitch not only got off with the temporary office manager, but also photocopied his privates at the office party, don't! Be magnanimous and urge the conversation in a different direction. You might have a great line prepared on how she had to use the enlarging option, but a quick point score isn't worth it in the long run. The same applies to pointing out mispronounced words and spilt drinks; be the person who asks the waitress for a napkin to help clean it up. And make sure, **when people do get it wrong, to give them a chance to make an honourable exit.** For example, if your boyfriend insists he knows the way to the hotel, don't squawk with laughter if he makes the wrong turn; ask if he thinks the other way might be quicker to give him a chance to make an elegant recovery. No one loves the company of a know-it-all who delights in telling them they are wrong.

never be an anteater

There are some masters of the genre though, who act like anteaters, **hoovering up any glory** where it is to be found. Their compliments sound like 'I love your dress – I have loads of that '80s retro hip' or 'I love this apartment – I'm making my place really minimal right now, too.'

You often know when you've been anteatered – usually you are about to say 'Thanks!' but then you're not sure if they have complimented you or themselves for their great taste/ intelligence/vision. The best way to avoid falling into this trap is to always make sure that you **GIVE credit, rather than TAKE it.**

You will do this naturally if you swap the 'I' for a 'you'.

'You look great in your '80s retro dress – you have great style.'

'You have made a great choice with these beautiful minimal pieces – what a lovely home you have created. I'm inspired.'

don't be a show-off – let them show off!

Everyone hates a show-off. Proving you are smarter, cooler and better connected than everyone else in your company is not a way to win yourself admirers. (You may, however, find yourself surrounded by sycophants, users and clinger-ons, having intimidated the nice regular folks or embarrassed yourself with the movers and shakers, who see you as a desperate small fry.) This doesn't mean, though, that you should dress in sackcloth and tug at your forelock like a medieval serf; you need to **learn to communicate your achievements and skills in an inclusive way.**

Finding common ground is the key. At a dinner party, you may find yourself talking about exercise with a fellow guest, giving you a chance to mention your passion for golf or the half marathon you've recently trained for (a 'discovered' achievement always seems more impressive than a brag). If they look disheartened, embarrassed to admit they haven't put on sportswear since school days, tell them how much training outdoors means to you, gently shifting the focus to a love of nature/the changing seasons, until you find something they can respond to. Once they start waxing lyrical about how much they love to see their garden at this time of year, bingo! You've found a subject they can happily expand upon, but also discovered some common ground – an essential part of why people trust one another. From then on you can talk about your different interests, having established in their minds that you are 'their kind of person'. **This technique will have a radically diverse mix of people all claiming you as fantastic.**

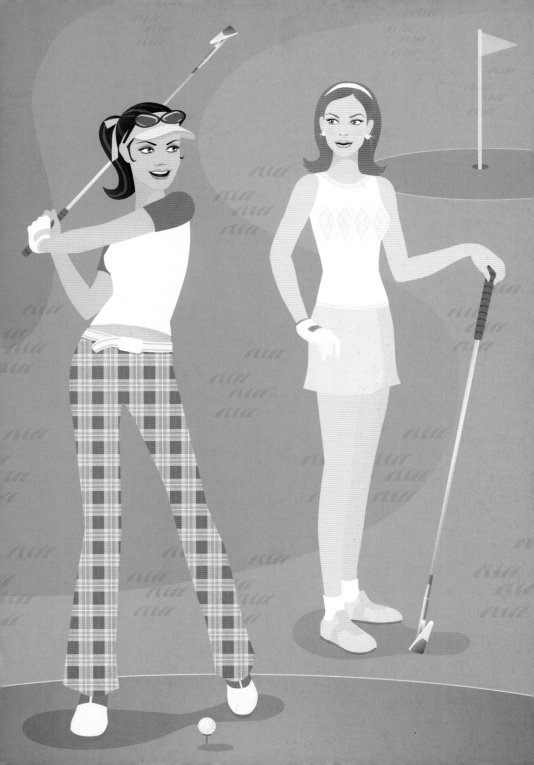

two minuses don't make a plus

No matter how careful and charming we may be, at some point **we all come across a negative person who is determined to be rude, aggressive or take anything you say the wrong way.** They are wilfully trying to infect you with their negativity or anger, and this is a situation which you should not try to 'win'. The best way to deal with someone in this circumstance is to stay vague. Should they rudely say, 'So how much do you earn?' and you don't want to answer, simply laugh and reply, 'Enough, thank you'. If they persist, repeat your line, and do so until they desist. Your aim here is not to win them over, but to keep your dignity in the face of their aggression. Others present will be able to draw their own conclusions, which will no doubt be that this person is hectoring and rude. And even if you think you can win a verbal battle of wits, **the truly elegant person doesn't want a victory over someone who is angry, sad or unhappy.** As well as adding to the general misery quotient in the world, it's a hollow victory and blows your appeal as a magnanimous and generous person.

never ask a closed question

Have you ever tried teasing someone out and got nowhere? Do two-word answers make you want to run and hide behind the curtains? The idea may be right, but the technique may need a little tweaking. **Don't ask 'closed questions' with no room for others to expand.** For example, 'Do you have any children?' might elicit the answer 'Four boys'. So follow up with an open-ended question with an elaboration point built in such as, 'Wow! I bet that's like having your own football team. They must run you ragged.' Which gives the other person a chance, and a reason, to expand upon the joys and challenges of having four sons.

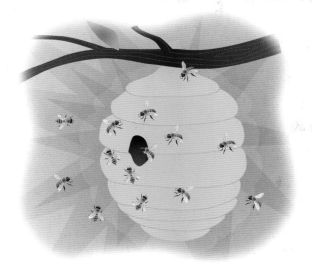

all bees, no honey

Have you ever found yourself in a new situation and been unsure what to do? Think of yourself as a bee or as a pot of honey (well, pollen to be exact, but it's not so pretty an image). Your action will prompt a reaction and you need to consider what would provoke the desired reaction. For example, you may think that asking your boyfriend to take the dry cleaning should be no big deal and it's his turn anyway, but knowing his usual resistance, you tense at the very thought of asking him, so your request comes out as stiff and aggressive. This will hit his competitive nerve, and he will bristle and begin coming up with reasons why he is just as busy as you are. Even if you are right, two bees will start buzzing angrily. You need to appeal to his attraction to honey; if you make the request explaining your early meeting and your crazy, busy day, and that it would be a real contribution and help, you will appeal to his protective nerve. Hey presto! Cleaning at the cleaners. Manipulative? No, just realistic. (Hey, I didn't design human nature.) You can apply this to anything: go in angry, you get angry; go in inquisitive and open, you'll get solutions.

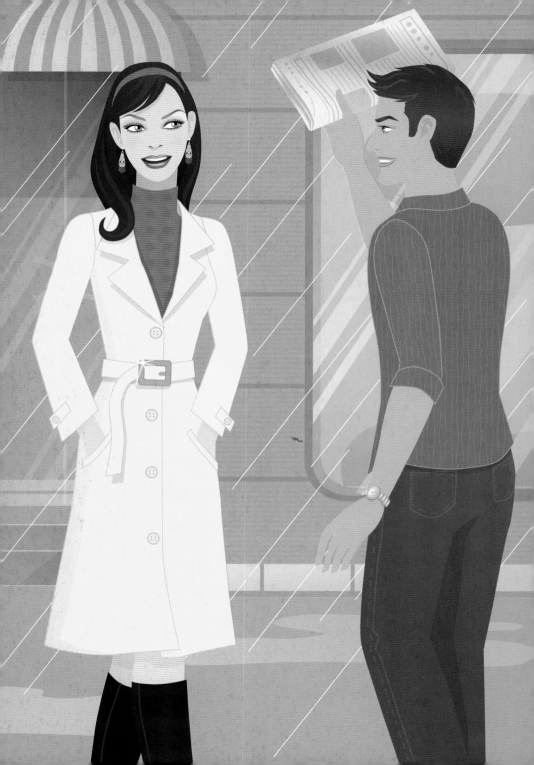

confidence building

> ❛ I've learned that you can tell a lot about a person by the way he/she handles these three things: a rainy day, lost luggage and tangled Christmas tree lights. ❜

Maya Angelou
(1928–), US poet and author

your **critical** *voice*

Being confident is pretty simple: it basically comes down to being your own best friend. We wouldn't tell our sister, mother or closest girl chum that they really shouldn't pick up a pan ever again after one burnt Sunday roast; that love will always elude them because that guy they didn't even really fancy didn't call them; or that the job interview they fluffed was their last chance of a career and they will end up living off out-of-date ready meals they found in the supermarket trash. So why, oh why, do women talk like that to themselves?

One of the key problems women can burden themselves with is a 'critical voice'. Most of us don't realize we do it, and think we are simply evaluating our own progress honestly or trying to 'buck up'. But this kind of behaviour can have far-reaching effects, holding us back from striving to achieve our goals (I'll never get that promotion) to making us miss chances when they appear (he's not looking at me, I look awful today). One of the most **refreshing and liberating** things to consider at this point is that, in reality, most people *aren't* looking at you. They *aren't* considering you, they *aren't* gossiping or pointing fingers because, as a rule, they have far too much stuff going on in their own lives, **namely themselves**, to really think about what's happening to you. So you can stop thinking your every gaffe and failure is burned onto other people's retinas. They're not, so get out there and try again.

'People may flatter themselves just as much by thinking that their faults are always present to **other people's minds,** as if they believe that the world is always contemplating **their individual charms and virtues.'**

Elizabeth Gaskell (1810–65), English novelist

positive
affirmation...

So stop talking dirty to yourself. Whenever you start an internal criticism, stop! Think about what you are saying and ask yourself if it has any truth, then ask yourself how you would feel if you let that belief go (Happier? Entering a room with a swagger rather than scuttling in under the radar like a beetle?). And sometimes we don't just do it in our heads, we say it out loud, too. One of the main problems women have lies in being their own PR. In an effort to connect with others, we sometimes use our flaws or weaknesses as a bonding device. But this can backfire messily, especially as we get older. Although no one wants to hang about with the super-perfect bitch, neither do they want to be dragging about a whiny bag of neuroses on a Friday night.

How you see the world affects how it sees you. If you think everyone is out to get you, you'll treat people as such and turn them off, making your projection a reality. You can spend all your time on a date putting your best foot forward but ruin the whole effect by blowing up at the waiter for bringing the wrong wine and muttering that it's typical of your bad luck. By the time you have rearranged your face back into the beatific smile you've presented to your date, there will only be a puff of dust where they turned on their heels and ran. If anything says **'high-maintenance nightmare', it's someone with no ability to let go of the little stuff.** Of course, no one likes a Stepford wife either, with a constant grin and a positive spin on everything; it just makes you seem simple-minded and possibly overmedicated. Once again, **the key is balance, but with an optimistic overview.**

cheating confidence

Research at the University of Ohio found that nodding
or shaking your head not only tells people what you are
thinking, but also influences how you feel. Nodding your
head up and down gives you confidence in the thoughts you
are having, whereas shaking your head undermines your
opinion to yourself. So, if you are telling someone you think
you would like to try singing lessons and could be good at
them, nod away; this will increase your confidence.

IF YOU FEEL like you're fluffing something up, YOU SHOULD look at the person opposite and realize they get it wrong sometimes, too. For every goal a top footballer scores, he has plenty of misses.

IF YOU FEEL disappointed at slow progress, YOU SHOULD break down your goal into simple steps and focus on each achievement as you edge towards the final result. A CEO of an international firm isn't born in a pinstripe babygrow, she works toward it. Same with athletes and musicians.

IF YOU FEEL panic starting to rise, YOU SHOULD focus on something like the desk or a lamp and start describing it to yourself; your brain can't get you into a tailspin if it's busy doing something. When you re-focus, you'll be much calmer.

IF YOU FEEL like you wish you were superconfident now, YOU SHOULD realize that confidence is better when it's built gradually with all the blocks firmly in place, so that if it gets knocked, it doesn't collapse. False confidence is just that; it looks very nice but won't stand up to closer examination.

homework

Be your own PR. First, you need to slay your demons, so write down the five
traits you have that are the most unhelpful or unattractive (complaining about
your weight, refusing to talk to new people at parties). Think about the reverse of
these situations, who you would be if you didn't do these things, and how to get
from one place to another. Is there anything you can physically do to transform
the situation? If you want a promotion at work but it would involve speaking in
public, can you ask to be sent on a training course that would address your fear?
Or could you try a kamikaze solution such as singing at the local karaoke club?

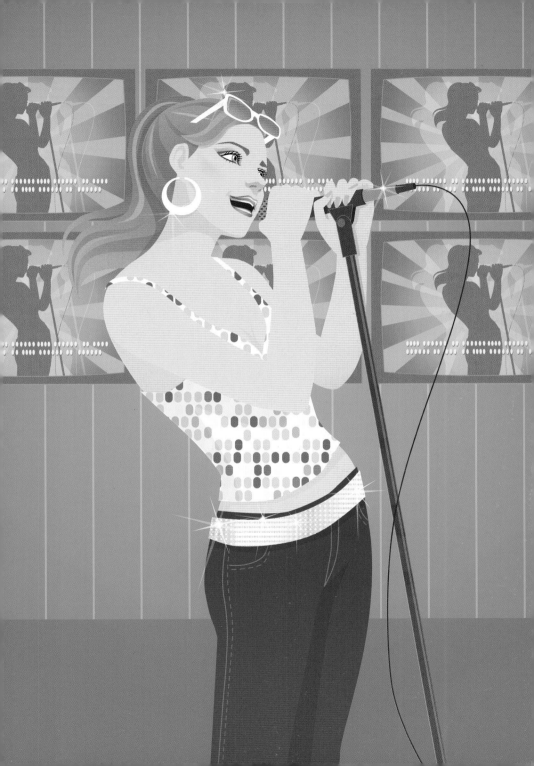

list five of your best qualities that you *should be* *playing up*

A good PR would never launch a new TV show by saying, 'It's such a fun programme but it's mainly due to the clever editing and the host is an awful drunk!' So why do you feel as if you must give all your attributes equal billing? Work out your strengths and play to them. If you are finding this difficult, entice a friend over with a bottle of wine and offer to do the same for her. If she says you are great at getting a party started, think about throwing a bash or offer to organize a weekend away with friends trying something new like white water rafting. Work out where your strengths lie and build on them, making them the focus of your energy and attention.

'**Develop interest in life** as you see it; in things, literature, music – the world is so rich, simply **throbbing with rich treasures,** beautiful souls and interesting people. **Forget yourself.**'

Henry Miller
(1891–1980), US author

put an end to
charm self-sabotage

Have you ever regretted saying something? The reality is that most of us have 'sensitive spots'. We can be charming as the sun is hot till the arrival of someone who plugs into our anxieties, and we find ourselves opening our big mouth and cringing at what comes out. **The best way to make sure that you are capable of acting like a queen in every situation is to be honest about your own insecurities,** so that you know when you might react badly. Do you ever find yourself engaging in a bit of unpleasant one-upmanship when you see the neighbour's new car, telling them you've signed up to receive the latest Lotus hot off the production line? Admit to yourself you are a bit envious.

Do you find yourself changing the subject when anyone talks about politics? **Accept you feel out of your depth.** Doing this means that when you see your neighbour you can compliment them on their lovely new car rather than get yourself in hock, making you both feel good. Admit you don't know much about politics and ask the person talking to elaborate rather than shut them down; your admission makes you come across as confident, plus you get the chance to learn something. **EVERYBODY WINS.**

And don't beat yourself up about it.
Everyone's personality is a mix of the nice and the not-so-nice; being a real grown-up is just about accepting that fact and controlling which stuff you put out into the world.

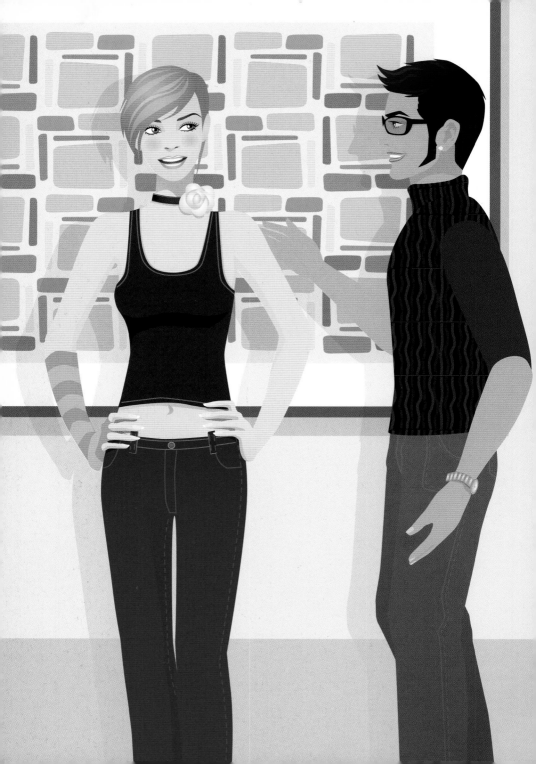

blushing: the confidence crusher

You've learned the patter, you're dressed to thrill and your hair is so glossy people are checking their lipstick in it. And then, as soon as you prepare to leap into the chat with your witty repartee, you feel that familiar flush. Lots of us do it, but we can still feel that blushing undermines all our hard work. So what do you do if it happens to you?

- Take a minute. Take three breaths in through the nose and out through the mouth (hide behind your glass a little if you feel self-conscious) and relax. Three breaths is all you need to change your state, taking you from nervous to natural.

- Realize that everyone has their 'thing'. If it's not blushing, it's sneezing; if it's not a funny habit of rubbing their nose, it's a verbal tick of padding their sentence with 'y'knows'. Only those with an agenda will draw attention or try to embarrass you because of it, and unless they are a gorgeous suitor teasing to get your attention, let them show themselves up for the crass meanie they are and let it go.

- Joke about it. Sometimes the best way to deal with such a circumstance is to draw attention to it yourself. It diffuses any awkwardness and is seen by most people as charming and self-effacing. Now if only you could learn to do it at will...

negative appeal...

Of course all this self-loathing affects the way we react to men. So what to do? Well, good news: men actually don't want you to be miserable and snivelling either. In fact, it positively turns them off.

The three authors – a lawyer, doctor and accountant – who wrote the book *What Men Want* busted lots of girls' myths about being nice. They claimed that we 'teach' men how to treat us, and if that's as a doormat, so be it. They also state that even the nicest guy will use a woman for sex, as a **'Wait-till-something-better-comes-along'** filler, simply to avoid being lonely. And it's up to us whether or not we sign up for this treatment.

bitch appeal

As soon as we start toddling as little girls, we begin to hear the word 'nice' with stunning regularity. 'That's not nice', 'Play nice', 'Be a good girl and be nice to your brother' (who just stole your bike/ate your sweets/pulled your hair). So we begin to rapidly connect in our minds the concept of 'nice' as essential to our popularity and desirability. That's great, if it stops you stealing the next-door neighbour's car, but let's get real: when did anyone ever say, 'I must shower her with diamonds/have her this instant/devote my life to making her mine 'cos she's just so darn nice!'

Sometime around adolescence, **we start to let this idea of pleasing everyone get us into trouble** and we find ourselves giving in to boys who pretend they may die of some kind of internal explosion due to spurned advances; or agreeing to wash the clothes of boyfriends who know where the launderette is; or lending money to a guy who promises to take us to dinner with it (sure, if 'Dinner' is running in the 4.15 at the racetrack), all because we are frightened of not being nice and saying 'no'.

Well, here's a news flash: **men aren't afraid of 'no'** – men *like* 'no'. A man who wants to truly be with you, and is a decent guy, either won't attempt this in the first place or will respect you more for firmly putting up the boundaries. It makes him feel he has found a prize and an equal worthy of his attention. So don't insipidly give in, hoping he'll realize he's being thoughtless – he won't give it a second thought (or you, for that matter). Which is why you shouldn't be surprised if you find yourself wailing as you find his dirty sock in your laundry two months after he left you, 'I can't believe he's going out with her, she's such a bitch!' She might be. And he probably likes it.

if you are never frightened,
you are probably dead

Fear is a natural part of living, as is making mistakes, losing a phone, putting on weight and arguing occasionally with your best friend. Finding your phone, losing a few pounds and getting drunk and taking stupid pictures with your best friend are also all part of the deal. Once you accept that and put an end to 'perfectionist syndrome' you will cope better with disappointments and setbacks.

It has been shown that the way people handle disappointments and setbacks is a clear indicator of how happy in general their lives will be. And there is no use hiding behind the belief that you are a pessimist or unlucky, or just have a bad temper. **Optimism and positivity can be learned at any time in your life,** so next time you start telling yourself it's the end of the world because you lost your phone, pause, laugh at yourself, then use another phone line to ring it. (Psychologists call this technique 'reframing', where you take the same set of facts and give them a different interpretation. Both ways of seeing it are 'true', but only one makes you happy.)

'Success is nothing more than spontaneous combustion. You must set yourself on fire.'

Reggie Leach
(1950–), Canadian hockey player

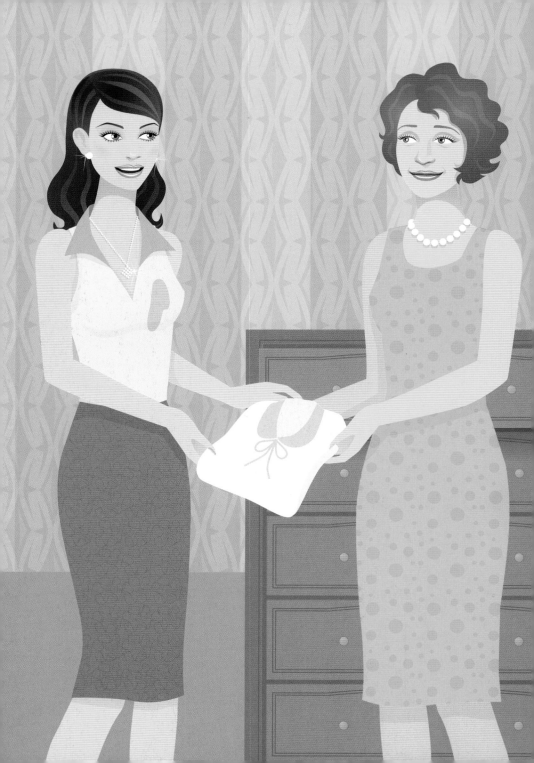

So how does the fear bit fit in? Well, we can also tell ourselves that feeling scared is a clear sign that we shouldn't be attempting something, are bound to fail or can't cope. But the **sensation of fear** (unless you are being chased by a bear through the woods) is usually just **telling you that something is important to you, that you want it badly and you will probably have to take a risk or stretch yourself to get it.** And if you never feel fear, either you never take a risk or you have never left the house. Neither one bodes well for your future.

dealing with the fear factor

Visualization can be incredibly helpful when tackling fear. First, position yourself comfortably in a straight-backed chair, hands resting lightly on your lap. **Become aware of your breathing, making it slow and measured.**

Imagine the situation that makes you the most anxious: meeting his parents for the first time, for example. Now imagine saying 'hello', going into the living room and accepting a cup of tea. Imagine accidentally spilling it all over yourself and their white sofa. What happens now? Your first instinct might be to run out of the house, screaming. Instead, **imagine laughing, admitting your horror and nerves, and bonding with his mum** while she finds you a new top to wear. See? No one ended up in prison.

Is there anything you can do before you begin? The best way to manage fear is to explode it. For example, if you're dreading the first day at work, try driving the route to make sure you won't be late and using the Internet to research the company ('we sell what to where again?').

Five instant ways to make
your confidence bulletproof

1 Be like a man. When you mess up, forgive yourself instantly. It wasn't intended to hurt or annoy, so why torture yourself? Unless you actually spent six months in your basement planning to bump into that old man or get your brother's new girlfriend's name wrong, what's the problem? (And if you did, you've got bigger problems than this one to worry about.)

2 Ask for more, and less. Next time something comes up that you want, like an exciting new account at work, ask to work on it. When a pile of extra work hurtles towards your team looking like its heading for your 'in' tray, insist it's shared. The news flash kept from most women is this: we get what we ask for, the squeaky wheel gets the oil and no one thinks you're worth the time off/extra cash until someone brings it to their attention – which means *you*. And another great secret: the more you ask, the easier it gets and the more you think you deserve it! Talk about an upward spiral…

3 See rejection as their loss. When the short, bald guy asks the fledgling model for her number and gets a knock-back, he doesn't go home and beg his mirror to reveal why no one loves him. He shrugs and tries the next stool. He might be the best lover, the most elegant orator or have millions stuffed under his mattress, whatever, he knows she's missing out. Whether it's true or not, it gives him the power to get back on the horse and try again (which is why you often see a short, bald guy with a pretty girl). If you don't get the job, you might have had an off-interview day or the interviewer may have had a thing about people with freckles. Who cares? Move on!

4 Be your own cheerleader. Don't ask someone if they think you can do it; say you can and then rise to the challenge (unless it's performing brain surgery). Then work like mad to make sure you do a great job.

5 Be clear about what you want. Don't be ashamed of ambition or desires; little girls aren't told it's OK to aim high so we think we should pretend middle is OK. But little girls don't want to buy expensive shoes or holiday in the Maldives…

'If you always do

what you've always done,

you'll always get

what you always got.'

From *Coming Back* by Ann Kaiser Stern,
US psychologist and author

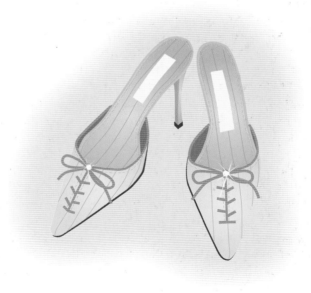

princess
ploy

Do you need a little ego boost but there's no one around to do it? Boyfriend's old news, parents are out of town, best friend's sick?

Be your own booster: get up five minutes earlier to make yourself some lovely fresh coffee; book yourself a pampering facial or splash out on some really expensive fabric conditioner to make your sheets smell delicious; buy a timer for your lamps so there's always a rosy glow to welcome you as you arrive home. **If you start believing you deserve life's little extras, you'll feel like it.** After all, a princess doesn't need a prince to come along and tell her she's a princess. **SHE'S ALREADY GOT A CROWN.**

how to appear
utterly confident...
even when things go wrong

You can actually use your mistakes to make yourself even more irresistible. For most people, there's nothing more tiresome than someone who is eternally perfect.

If you make a gaffe, trip up the stairs or drop a drink, have the elegance to catch the eye of the stranger desperately looking away to save your blushes. A hearty guffaw will break the tension, making everyone around you grateful. Assuming it wasn't a serious accident (in which case laughing is probably not the best option), what's the worst thing that can happen? You scrape a knee or have to replace a broken mug. **It's not worth ruining your mood for the rest of the day.** Still not convinced? Haven't you seen those Meg Ryan movies where she does something 'kooky' like walking into a door and seems utterly irresistible and cute? Recover well with good humour and being clumsy could end up a serious weapon in your charming arsenal.

Attitude determines altitude, how high you will fly in life.'

Patricia Russell-McCloud,
US motivational speaker and author

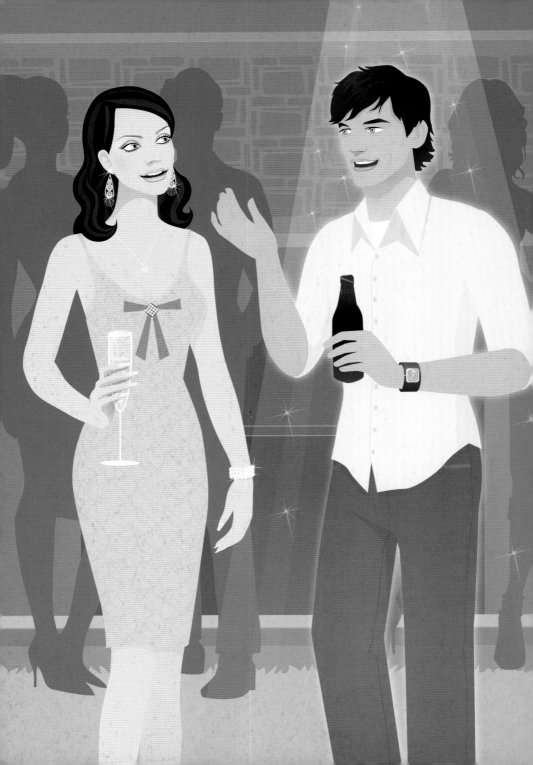

the charm offensive

7

> ' I'm convinced that it's energy and humour. The two combined equal charm. '
>
> **Judith Krantz**
> **(1928–), US novelist**

what to say and do in
critical situations

Knowing what to say when it really counts is always tough to do, and most people's biggest worry. You can make sure your interview suit or party dress is pristine, practise your beaming smile for hours in front of the mirror, but what you can't do is hand the other person a script of what you would like them to say, unfortunately.

Hell, who wants that anyway? The key to getting it right is to look on it as a game, and the irresistible woman sees it as a chance to rise to a challenge and think on her feet. But while you are getting to that **'happy-to-fly-by-the-seat-of-my-pants'** stage, here's a few nuggets for your bag of tricks.

In any situation, the key is to sniff the air. A common mistake for women is a kind of 'They should love me for who I am!' defensiveness. Actually, no. The charming person knows that it's not all about them. You need to gauge the tone from the people around you, then make a decision. If, when meeting the boyfriend's parents, they want to keep things formal at first, don't start cracking rude jokes to the dad and ask the mum where she buys her underwear. **You may think your kookiness is endearing, but it's not: it's just alienating.** Let them set the pace and when they are comfortable, you can start to influence it. Boundaries exist for a reason; trample on them at your peril.

Going with the flow also gives you time to work out a few things. Taking a strong position from the start can alienate. Ordering a round of drinks for everyone might seem the behaviour of a charmer, but it can fall flat if it turns out you've crashed an Alcoholics Anonymous party. **Someone truly charming responds to other people, rather than demands the limelight at all costs.** Remember, it's how you make people feel that counts, and that has more to do with your delivery and body language in the first few lines of conversation.

parties

Parties are great because they always have a host. So **ask them to introduce you to the people you want to meet.** If they can't be found, use their absence as a way to meet that person anyway, by simply asking, 'Hi, do you know where Susan is? I wanted to know if there is any mineral water.' Even if they have no idea, you are at least making an exchange. Assuming Susan isn't at your side with a bottle of mineral water (even if she is, the irresistible woman should be able to laugh at herself), you can always ask how they know the host, all of which is a nice and gentle way of keeping the conversation moving while you hit them with your winning body language.

meeting the parents

When we really like another person, meeting his parents can become an agonizing event in our minds, the importance of which we often blow up into huge proportions. We can often feel that if we fail, it could mean the end of our relationship and a life spent getting old with a roomful of cats in a rundown part of town. Er, no, it's actually just tea. **The main objective here is simply to get the parents of your man to decide that you are suitable.** All they want to know, at this early stage, is that you are clean, don't eat with your feet and are nice to their offspring. This is a getting-to-know-you session, a gentle introduction to see what it's all about, so you don't need to sing, impress them with your tap dancing skills (especially if you haven't got any), or show them your driving licence. If you can leave them with a small glow of warmth, all the better.

When you meet, give them a firm handshake (placing a second hand over theirs is a winning technique that politicians use to communicate warmth) and give a bright 'Hello, Mr and Mrs...'.

Never use first names unless invited to do so. **It is their privilege to bestow family niceties upon you, welcoming you in,** so calling his mother 'Babs' before she's even asked you to call her 'Barbara' will just make them feel like you are being pushy (you are) and will encourage them to pull back (which they should).

Try to find common ground. If they are country dwellers, don't tell them how (because you hate being away from the city for too long) you've started sucking on car exhausts. This will make them feel they have to justify their choices to you and put you on opposing teams. Instead find things you do like – an obvious one being their son. You can ask to see pictures, or for stories or anecdotes, and they will usually light up like a Christmas tree at the chance of reliving his Scouts parade. **There is only one thing mothers like to talk about more than themselves, and that's their kids.** Obvious etiquette rules apply: don't get drunk at dinner unless they do, don't pat Dad's butt to be cheeky, and most of all, don't grill Mum for details of his ex: you can save all that for meeting two.

job interview

Body language plays a big part in this scenario, as head hunters, managers and recruitment officers often look for non-verbal signs, knowing that verbally speaking, candidates are going to be putting their best foot forward and fudging a few facts. And even if it is a job you aren't sure that you want, make sure that, on the interview front, you give it a gold medal performance. Every practice run will make you better for the job interview you've been waiting for.

You will be judged as soon as you arrive. **Be early, even if it means you have to hang around in a coffee shop for half an hour.** It's almost impossible to recover from a panicked late start and you will immediately project anxiety. Don't re-read notes while in the waiting room: read a magazine or look around in a relaxed, composed fashion. Make sure you know the names and job titles of those interviewing you. When they are ready to see you, don't peek round the door asking if you can come in, stride purposefully and with confidence. They are ready to see you or you'd still be sitting outside, so don't dither.

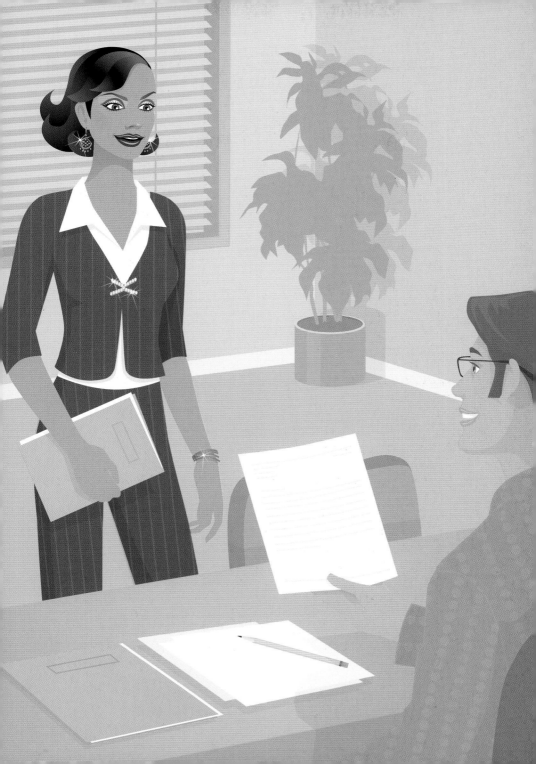

A recent study showed that an opinion formed in 20–32 seconds of a taped interview (essentially the introduction phase) by non-professional viewers of a candidate matched the rating of self-assurance and likeability very closely to that of a professional interviewer after they had spent a further 20 minutes with them. So basically, **this critical 'here I am' stage counts. A lot.**

When you meet your interviewer, make sure your handshake counts. No longer just a macho stand-off tool, research has shown that a firm handshake on a woman makes a huge difference to how they are viewed. **It shows they have confidence and are assertive, making them desirable candidates.** When it comes to choosing a seat, if it's not obvious, don't ask. Select a seat opposite the interviewer and avoid a squishy sofa from which it's hard to get up – an inelegant flash of the knickers and a wobble on your new heels as you try to emerge from a squeaky low-level couch can unravel even the most polished interview. And it's not exactly the parting shot you want to leave uppermost in their minds.

Keep eye contact with your interviewer. If there is more than one, look at them in turn and emphasize points with assertive hand gestures (that doesn't include punching the air). **Keep a respectable distance physically and don't be pally or use slang or over-familiar terms; it's a big professional no-no.** Clenching your hands and tapping your foot is like wearing a big badge saying, 'Hi, I'm nervous'. Try not to do it.

'Good luck is when preparation meets opportunity.'

Seneca (4BC–AD65), Roman philosopher

Although you may have certain verbal tics (uhhmm, ahhh, speaking in a nervous squeaky voice under pressure), don't try to be artificially cocky or assured. **Your voice should change as you get excited or passionate about an area, you should smile where appropriate,** but not wear the constant rictus smile of the recently deceased. A natural flow in tone and expression shows confidence and trustworthiness. If you tend to blather or panic, do a mock interview with a friend beforehand so you feel more prepared and have talked out some of the junk. It helps you recognize the salient points and log them in your mind for the big day.

Reading the interviewer's body language is also essential. Nodding as you speak is a sign of encouragement and means they like what you are saying or want you to carry on expanding upon your theory. Tilting their head or leaning forward means they are listening closely and are interested; keep talking.

If they are fiddling, drumming their fingers, folding their arms or leaning away, they are disinterested or don't agree, so change tack or wrap it up so they can ask you something else. When it's time to say goodbye, initiate a handshake (making sure you have left a clean, crumple-free resumé), hold their gaze and smile at each interviewer in turn. **Then go home and collapse into the nervous wreck you really are.**

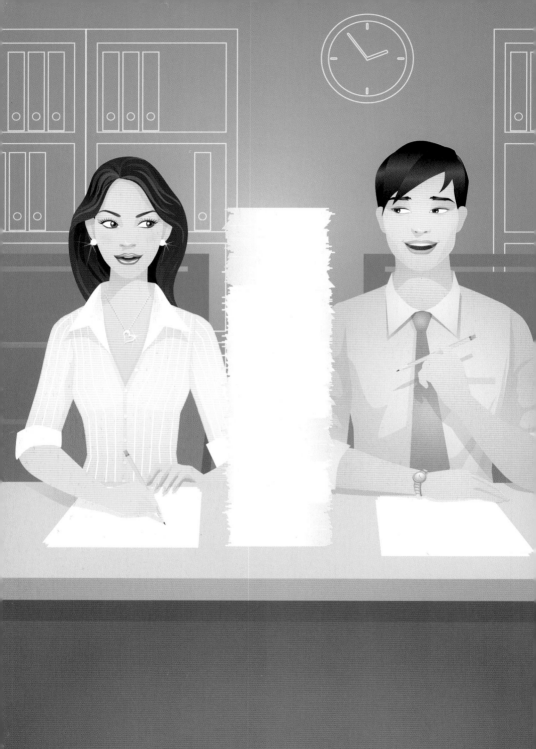

first day at work

Great, you wowed the interviewers and got the job. The key now is to make the transition to your new workplace as stress-free and easy as possible.

The first thing to remember is that you will quite likely have no real idea about why the previous incumbent of your role left. They could have been headhunted or sacked, and there may be a residue of ill feeling or a 'no one could replace Marjorie' attitude from your new colleagues. But the only thing you can do is to wait and see. The first layer of information may be from the disgruntled office gossip or the junior who was hoping to get your position. Here, the best thing is to be friendly, but firm. Don't get drawn into any allegiances early on. Many a 'helpful' after-work drink has turned out to be the forays of an office Lothario. **Ask a lot of friendly questions, appealing to people's expertise, and be appreciative of any help and information.** Then watch and learn.

work etiquette

While no one likes a yes woman, not everyone hates their boss either: neither ingratiating yourself with the seat of power or trying to win lunch chums with impressions of your manager's silly walk will win you allies. Keeping your opinions to yourself is a safe option, particularly as an 'on paper' hierarchy often counts for little and it takes time to work out the real allegiances. The biggest egos aren't always the ones with the biggest pay packets, and you may have more to fear from the PA to your boss than the head of marketing, so bruise others at your peril. Some simple advice is to give others the benefit of the doubt, don't get too emotional, be polite in manner and concise in language, and steer clear of giving negative criticism – always try to put a positive spin on any feedback you give.

the charm offensive 137 ☆

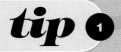

the emergency cover-all: never be speechless

There are times when we all hit the communication wall. We are tired, we've had a rotten day and we just can't produce that special zing to be the belle of the ball. Or maybe we're just hungover. **But the great thing about devising a charm offensive is that it gives you a coping strategy for any situation that may arise;** all you have to do is show up and let your preparation, as it were, do the talking.

Your palms are sweating, your heart is beating, and your mind is blank. So forget talking. **What you need to do here is to get the focus away from yourself while you gather your thoughts.** The best way to do this is by paying the other person a compliment that includes a question. As with all compliments, make sure it is rooted in genuine truth. Find something pleasant, and don't just say 'Wow, what a lovely scarf' because they can easily say 'thank you', and that's the end of that. To compensate you'll end up coming up with a list of other nice things to say, which will make you sound like a stalker. Instead say something like, 'What a great colour that scarf is on you. Is it cashmere/a present/bought locally?' This gives them lots to respond to, such as, 'I love the colour pink – I think it lifts my hair colour' or 'It's actually silk and so soft – it was a gift from my husband last Christmas' or 'I bought it in India when I took a three-month sabbatical.' **This technique works on several levels from making them feel good, showing you are paying attention to them and revealing lots of new areas where the conversation could go.**

This trick can be sustained for a while. Use communications expert Liel Lowndes' technique of parroting. **Simply repeat the last few pertinent words to the other person to keep them flowing.** Say you are talking about the dress code for a work dinner with a colleague:

HER: 'I think it's sort of cocktail party smart.'
YOU: 'Cocktail party?'
HER: 'Yes, you know, eveningwear but not too showy.'
YOU: 'Not too showy?'
HER: 'Uhuh. I'm thinking maybe a black dress I got for my sister's wedding. It has long sleeves.'

They won't even notice your lack of contribution to the conversation, as they are happily in their own reverie.

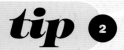

tip ❷

everyone could do with some extra lovin'

Remember the days when you were in long socks and your mother made you stay in to write a thank-you card to your gran, or hinted that she preferred a homemade card rather than a shop-bought one for a birthday? At the time such things seemed like a deadly chore, and the glow it gave to the recipient barely a blot on your radar. Well, you're not seven any more, so buy yourself some nice note paper and a set up a calendar reminder on your computer. **Taking the time to jot a short card to say thanks for a great weekend, or to send a birthday card that arrives on time, will gain you credit in the Royal Bank of Charm.** See it as a debit credit system: goodwill stored up throughout the year will stand you in good stead when you have to make a withdrawal, such as asking for the receipt to exchange that dreadful reindeer sweater from Aunt Phyllis.

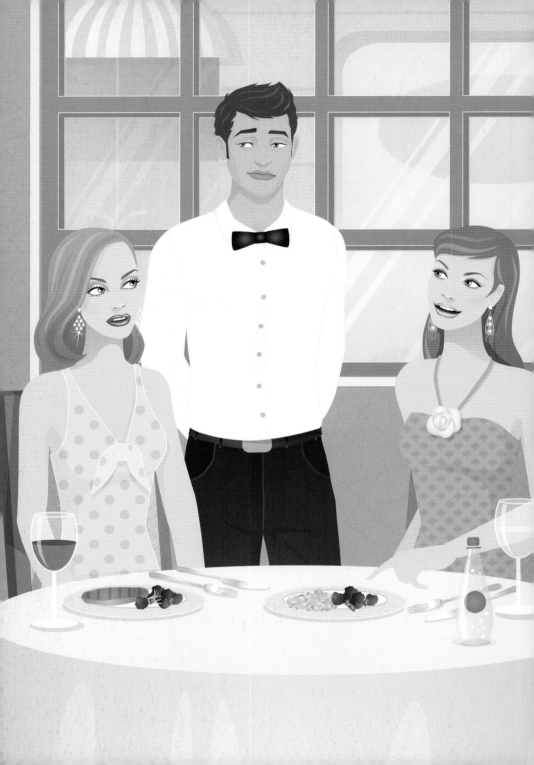

handling the *hard stuff* 8

'Life's challenges are not supposed to paralyze you, they're supposed to help you discover who you are.'

Bernice Johnson Reagon
(1942–), US composer and songleader

Of course, by now we can all skip, sparkling, through a party or turn a neutral situation into a winning one. It's the tough stuff, however, that can cause a chink in our charm armour. And managing to turn around a possibly destructive situation by not just coming off OK, but coming off as liked? Now that's the sign of a true charm Jedi master...

'There is no such thing as a problem without a gift for you in its hands. You seek problems because you need their gifts.'

Richard Bach
(1936–), US author

how to tell the *boss* *she's wrong*

Sounds impossible? Well, handled properly it can be done and can even add to your credibility in the workplace. When approaching this sticky situation, make sure that you:

 Are prepared. Don't waste her – or his – time by wandering in with a half-formed plan and no real ideas. Get the facts to back up your argument and even write them down if you have to. This shows you know your boss is a force to be reckoned with.

 Do it in private. Don't laugh or disagree with an idea in front of the rest of the team or your boss may cut you down just to prove a point, even if your idea was the best thing since someone thought of combining 'Twister' with alcohol.

 Talk it up. Don't say another idea is all bad; say what you liked first, so that you seem to be starting from a point of agreement.

 Be prepared to hear no, and be polite about it. A missed opportunity is a shame but the world won't stop spinning; a slanging match with your superior is hard to recover from.

 Be ready to accept with good grace if your boss brings you into a project later. She may not have gone for your first idea, but a good presentation, initiative and respect are all things any boss needs more of. If you are asked to contribute ideas next time, don't be bitter, thumbing your nose and saying, 'Told you it was the right thing!', just see it as the foot that got the rest of you in the door.

make a *pulling pact*

Single women love to go out and talk to each other in great depth about the lack of good men available, how they never get chatted up, whether they will die alone eaten by their cats... To any remotely interested guy watching from the sidelines, two female heads bent over in impassioned chat, bodies turned towards each other, hands flailing, mouths moving a mile a minute – you may as well have strapped on two no-entry signs.

You may both look stunning and a million men may be interested in you but no one will ever come close enough to find out the real irresistible you. Because despite what your mouths say, your actions say **GO AWAY**. Instead of conveying the charm you intend, **you appear standoffish** and completely unapproachable.

Of course, **good friends are essential to women's mental health.** Studies show women live longer, more happily and have less instances of serious illness because of the wonderful effects of the loving social networks we create for ourselves. And no woman worth her girl stripes will turn her back on a friend who needs to rant and rave about the boss/ex-boyfriend/interest rates on her mortgage. But you also have to be realistic. Agree on a '**pulling pact**' so that should Mr Right make his interest known, you can return the wink.

pulling pact rules

⭐ **If your friend has a serious worry they want to discuss in private with no interruptions, go to a quiet restaurant for dinner or an out-of-the-way bar so you can give her the undivided attention she needs before heading to a more social venue later.**

⭐ **Agree to a game of two halves. Given the chance, we can all offload our worries for hours on end, but give each other a 'whinge' hour, then agree to change the subject. As well as being considerate to the other's needs, it will help you put the worries to one side for a time.**

⭐ **If you see someone you like, you can have a 'time out' to go and chat. Agree together what you are comfortable with. Fifteen minutes is long enough to work out if you want to exchange numbers and meet the guy at a later date.**

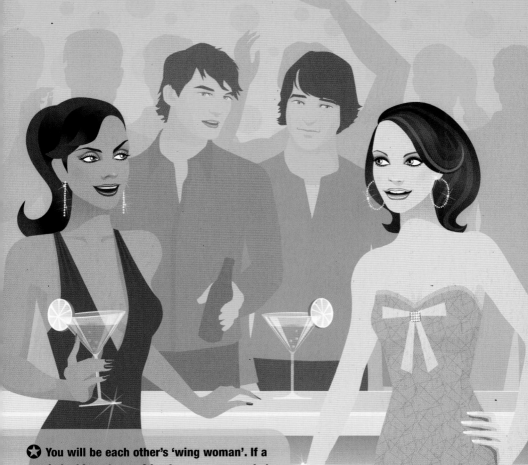

⭐ You will be each other's 'wing woman'. If a guy is looking at your friend, you may even help along the meeting process. It's so much easier to be bold when you aren't facing rejection.

⭐ No matter how enamoured/ drunk you are, you should never desert each other – make sure you both get home safely. If he really liked you on Saturday, he'll really like you on Sunday when you chat on the phone. (Plus it helps prevent any ill-advised liaisons.)

charming the *charmless*

Some people are so negative, draining and self-obsessed that it may seem impossible to charm them, but sadly, it's also sometimes impossible to dump them because they may be your boss, mother or even best friend. These people take a special kind of handling.

how to win them over...

First, you just won't win by going head to head with these people. They are trying to pass the misery and anger around so they feel less alone; this means they will seek out every opportunity to start a fight or act like the injured party, so forget a frank and open exchange of views (unless it's a relationship you truly value and you want to start afresh). Here, you should aim to **get in, get what you need and get out.**

The key to getting your evil boss to give you the Friday off you desperately need is not to suck-up or plead (the truly irresistible woman keeps her dignity intact at all times). Rather, you should be looking for ways around her defences. **Try one, or all of the following winning tactics.**

it's your decision

Instead of saying 'I need Friday off', say 'Do you think the department can cope without me on Friday?', thus putting the **emphasis on *your boss's* needs, not yours.**

the empathy ploy

If your boss complains she is overworked already, **soothingly acknowledge her plight** rather than pointing out she has just been out for a two-hour hair appointment. 'I know how much you have to do right now, which is why I'll have that report on your desk before I leave, so it's to hand if you need it.'

show your appreciation

When she agrees to give you the day off, make sure you say a polite and firm thank you. It is your right to have time off, so you don't need to grovel backwards out of the room, but **make sure you acknowledge the gesture.**

the happy spin

In the face of negativity, you will gain extra points with the moaner if you can leave her feeling better than she did before you arrived. If your boss says she is annoyed about being so busy, sympathize with her stress, then point out that she is so key to the running of things that she's a victim of her own success. Then focus on something upcoming that is enjoyable – a big office party or the Christmas holidays. **Refocusing someone on the good stuff leaves your boss with a warm glow** that will be associated with you. And you get Friday off.

get someone to apologize to you

Something went wrong. Your boss wants your head on a stick and is storming towards your desk to fetch it. Just remain calm. **Don't butt in, don't start apologizing, just listen.** Then immediately acknowledge the mistake by saying, 'I understand how frustrating it must have been that the computer died halfway through the presentation. I should have packed an extra battery – I'm sorry.' Your boss will probably be startled that you were willing to accept the blame and, having anticipated a wrangle, will immediately calm down. More often than not they will say, 'Oh, well, yes it was annoying, but I suppose it wasn't the end of the world.' Don't dither, apologize again: 'I am very sorry though, it was my mistake.' Before you know it, your boss will end up saying, 'Oh, heck, it can happen to anyone. Don't worry about it any more. I should have checked myself, too.' **And that's the end of it. Hurrah!**

TIP: do you want to be right or happy?

For some people, it's the same thing, but for most of us it's a good way to get our perspectives right. You may know that the person who just nipped in your parking spot is wrong, but will a full-scale argument improve your day or leave you feeling even more angry? If they know they're doing it, they're probably looking for someone to vent on (somehow angry people always get in more run-ins than the rest of us). If they really didn't see you, it's up for debate, so what the hell? But a great way of working out where to put your energy is to apply the 'pick your battles' logic. You can't win 'em all, so save your resources for the ones that count.

telling someone off at work

Sometimes being a boss is hard, especially when your heart and your head don't match. Say you have a member of staff who comes in late every morning. She looks tired and irritable most of time. **Here's what you do.**

You ask her into your office and tell her you have noticed her tardiness and would like to know what the problem is. She explains her mother is sick and she needs to pop in every morning to take her breakfast. Show sympathy, recognizing that it is difficult for her to meet all her demands. You then explain your situation: that other staff have noticed and they are starting to imagine lateness is allowed; that they are either disgruntled about arriving on time while she flouts the rules or they are following her lead. You would like to avoid issuing her with a formal warning, but need to follow company policy.

This next bit is the most important. **You ask her how you both can solve this dilemma.** Explain you understand her difficulties, but you also need to send a clear message to the others. If she stares at you blankly, come up with a suggestion, such as that you agree between you that, for a limited period, she has a later start and finish period and that this is communicated to the other employees. She may propose taking a shorter lunch hour to make up the time. Either way, **she is part of the solution.** She will also feel relieved you are acknowledging her problem and supporting her as best you can.

saying sorry

The best thing when you have to bite the bullet and apologize, is to do it simply and without excuses. Offered up quickly and willingly, an apology is much more effective than one that is dragged out and a bit lame.

complain with class

There are two important things to remember when complaining: first, **if you start off shouting you have nowhere left to go;** second, try to preserve your humanity.

ON THE PHONE: In these times of call centres and multimanagement levels, often the person who receives your complaint is rarely the one responsible for the error. And if their job is basically to field the calls of angry and disappointed people, well, you can imagine what their day is like. So treat them as a professional and with courtesy if you want a similar response. As you can see time and time again on nature programmes, going in with a hostile angle will ensure that you are met with one. Be warm and show a little empathy. Have a notepad handy to ask for the person's name and jot down any points that might be important. If you aren't getting anywhere, ask for their advice on the best procedure to follow, and if they are resolutely blocking you, politely ask to speak to a supervisor or have head office details.

IN A RESTAURANT: Only the very weak and very angry take out their power trips or frustrations on a waiter. On the charmless scale it holds the number-one spot with chewing your toenails in public. When something is wrong, a warm smile and simple statement of fact is enough to get your point across. If you feel the apology/replacement is not as placatory as you would like, mention it without hostility, see what is offered and, if necessary, ask if you can see the manager. If your waiter's face falls, it is often a good time to reassure them that you are happy with everything they have done, but appreciate they might be following a company policy you don't agree with. This kind of behaviour is more likely to garner you a free bottle of wine than someone spitting in your soup in the kitchen.

Whatever happens, **never get personal.** As soon as you do this, any ground you may have won will be lost as the shutters come down. Besides, it just makes you look mean if they're nice, and lets them know they got to you (their version of winning), if they're not.

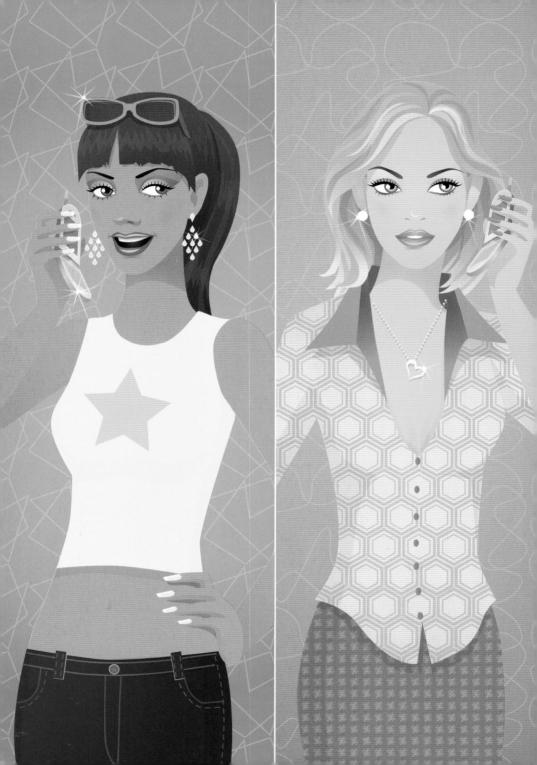

bring a friendship back from the edge

So you're both annoyed. You both think you are right and the irritated tone of voice and the abrupt phone call have you both furious and on the edge of calling it a day. When women fight, just as when we love, **things can get pretty heated, pretty fast.** Before you know it, frustrations and anxieties have built up on both sides with such speed that you're totally at each other's throats. **So how can you claw it back?**

Simply, put the claws away. Even if you think it may be too late, go and see your friend one last time, put your hand on her arm and say, 'Listen, kid, we've been Sarah and Susan for lots of years now and I'm sure that this isn't going to be the end of us. Like the boob tube fight of '84 almost was.' Reminding someone of all the good stuff will give you both a chance to remember why you are so upset in the first place: because you mean a lot to each other.

If you can stand to do it there and then, each have a 20-minute turn to get stuff off your chest. If you can't, suggest you meet up in a week/month to have a chat but make sure your parting words are warm. **Everyone is allowed to mess up and one bad incident shouldn't overshadow years of good ones.**

And if it can't be resolved? Wave goodbye graciously and stay tight-lipped to the gossips. Some fellow travellers in this life were only meant to be with us for part of the journey. Remember the good stuff and **don't dwell on the bad: it will only stop you from trusting and making new friends.**

quit your job
so they want you to stay

When it comes to leaving a job, most of us don't leave the one we have unless we think we would be happier elsewhere. Which may beg the question, who needs to leave the door open? But with the current climate of short contracts and freelance work, and just the slim possibility that perhaps your new position won't be as comfortable as you had hoped, **it's a good idea to leave things on the best possible terms.** And you'll always want a good reference. Not to mention the fact that even if your boss was a sociopath who made your waking hours a living hell, they might not necessarily be the boss forever. Make sure you don't leave a big black mark on your personnel file and you'll have a better chance of returning to the fold should you wish to in the future.

So how do you pull off this feat? Well, it's a case of using your charm to **put a honey gloss on all you say.**

- **Don't say that you couldn't wait to leave and have approached everyone you could think of, using the company phone, for the last six months and are accepting half your current salary just to get out of there. Instead say you were approached (if it's too much of a stretch, say you went for the new position as it offered you a chance to expand your skills and bank balance) and feel it's too much of an opportunity to miss.**

- **Offer to help find your replacement and work out a handover period or dossier to ease the transition.**

- **Don't take anything more than what you came with. A pocket full of pens, a stolen client – these may all seem like fair game, but have far-reaching effects on how people see you.**

- **Make sure you know your facts so that you don't miss out on any time-related bonus (like leaving two weeks before Christmas). If you have holiday to use up, work out if you want to reduce your notice period or take the money. Decide what you want in advance so you can request it when you hand in your notice.**

- **Don't tell everyone you work with how glad you are to move on: you'll just make them feel bad and they'll resent you, and who knows where they'll turn up again? In the same spirit, make sure you do your work properly to the last.**

- **If you don't state the reason for leaving as bad treatment, don't use it in your exit interview. You will look mealy-mouthed and they are not interested in losing another employee to protect one who has already left.**

- **In your official notice letter make sure you give your boss a boost. Mention the enjoyable experience it has been working for this company, under the good tutelage of 'X' and you hope that there may be a chance to renew your professional relationship with the company in the future. This is going to be kept on file so it's good to leave on the best note possible. And after all, handle it properly, and they might even encourage you stay. Now that's an exit!**

get your partner to listen to you without rolling his eyes

With men, timing is very important. If you are poised behind the door waiting to perform a verbal assault about how you need more help with the kids, you can rest assured he'll try to drown you out with the sound of the TV. You will both sit in separate parts of the house wondering, 'Why can't I just get a little bit of understanding? What's wrong with a little bit of empathy?'

Both of you really need some time to decompress.

Let him have half an hour watching the TV or doing homework with the kids and then ask if you can make some time to talk something through. This isn't about getting permission, it's about respecting someone else's needs and energy stores. You can even offer a trade-off: half an hour each to let off steam (this also stops you from falling into the trap of your partner just becoming a dumping ground for your woes and nothing else). If he looks pained, tell him you can talk it through at the weekend if that works better. **Giving him the option will make him feel less beleaguered** and we all appreciate this consideration. Chances are he'll then make a suggestion to talk later that day or the next morning. It can also help if you spell out what you need from him. If you say, 'Honey, I just want to drink a glass of wine and fill you in on my day', he will understand you just want to deliver your thoughts to him and he isn't expected to do anything about it. But if you want help from him, ask him outright. Don't change tack halfway through, then get frustrated when he just nods, thinking you still want him to be in good listener mode. For example, say, 'I don't know what to do about changing my shifts at work. How would you handle it?' **If you stick to time limits and be clear about what you want, you will find him increasingly receptive to these types of chats.**

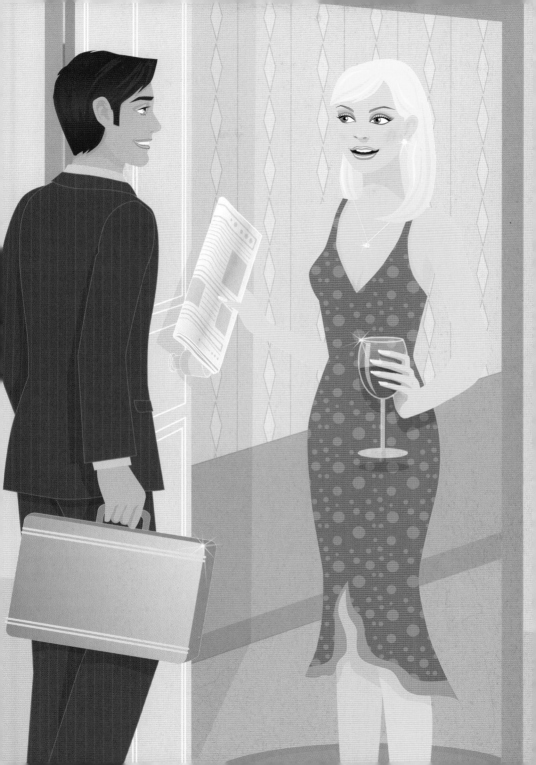

send condolences

When someone dies, often there seems very little solace you can offer to those left grieving. It's one of life's most difficult situations to acknowledge, but acknowledge it you must. **Many people mention how grateful they were for condolences after the event.** The first action to take is to send a note or card, or, if appropriate, to call. With a phone call, never ask for details unless they are offered, but do ask if they need any help or support. With a note, say something specific about the person and how they touched your life. And should you bump into the bereaved, make sure you take a moment to talk to them. **Part of the trauma of grief is the isolation,** so even if you don't get much of a response, you are helping in some tiny way.

turning around a hostile room

There's a problem with a group of people; it could be staff, residents or members of a social club. If you are in charge of sorting out the problem, there are a few general techniques that will help you placate the group and allow you to reach a decision in a calm environment. For example, as an area manager, you are sent to speak to a regional office of belligerent and furious staff, all of whom have a lot to say and intend to say it. You immediately feel defensive and want to take a strong stance against the criticism that is bound to be levelled at you. How can you go from being seen as the management's pawn, to a trusted confidante and even a friend?

Initially take no position. Ask if you can have a room in which to talk to people on a one-on-one basis and invite people to do just that. Tell them you want to understand the situation fully and invite them to offload their concerns. Make notes, smile, be open and respectful, and don't get into arguments. **Just listen.**

When you have heard everyone, speak to the group as a whole and let them know you have listened to their concerns, realized the common threads and understand their worries. It may be that the company line has already been decided, or that you have gathered more information that could be useful in the decision-making process. **Either way, giving people the chance to air their fears and pitch their case will immediately dissipate hostility.** Then, when you return with the decision, you will be welcomed with respect and openness, rather than resentment.

AND FINALLY... *be the guest*
everyone wants to RSVP

Now you know all about being charming. The tricks, the signals, the quirks, the style. You have the ability to influence the opinions formed by those around you, even in the briefest of meetings. But there is one trick left that will tip the balance in your favour, so you become the must-invite guest to any type of gathering.

Think of how you felt when you first started reading: unsure and convinced there was a social code you were missing, taking any rejection personally as a sign of failure. Now imagine everyone else in the room and, from your new position of strength, **start extending the hand of inclusion.** See that woman hovering by the sign-in desk at the work conference? Ask her a question which invites her into the group. What does she think of the report just released? What is her connection with the event? At parties, catch the eye of anyone you meet getting a drink – smile, make a quip and ask how they know the host. Most of these people will see you as a welcome saviour from their own uncertainty; others will regard you as confident and astute. Without doubt, all of them will find you utterly charming. You have become the social glue that brings everyone together. **Welcome to being an irresistible woman!**

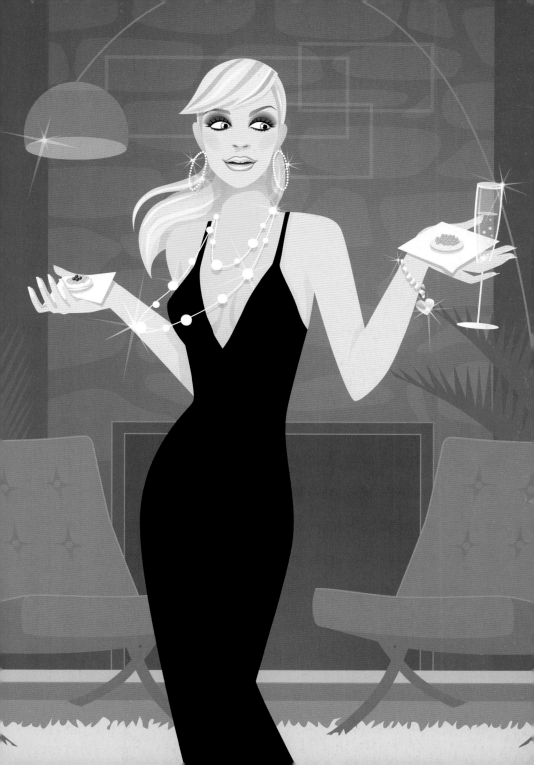

resources

Argov, Sherry, *Why Men Love Bitches,* Adams Media Corporation, 2002.

Cabot, Tracy, *How to Make a Man Fall in Love with You,* Dell Books, 1984.

Demarais, Anne and White, Valerie, *First Impressions: What You Don't Know About How Others See You*, Bantam, 2004.

Friedman, Dr Sonya, and Deswaan, C.B., *Take It From Here: Growing Up, Getting Real and Moving On*, Kensington Publishing, 2004.

Gerstman, Bradley, Pizzo, Christopher and Seldes, Rich, *What Men Want: Three Professional Single Men Reveal to Women What It Takes to Make a Man Yours*, Quill (HarperCollins), 2000.

Glass, Lillian, *I Know What You're Thinking: Using the Four Codes of Reading People to Improve Your Life*, John Wiley & Sons, 2002.

Helmanis, Lisa, *Master Dating*, Infinite Ideas, 2005.

Holden, Robert, *Success Intelligence*, Hodder Mobius, 2005.

Kasl, Charlotte Davis, *If the Bhudda Dated*, Penguin, 1999.

Lowndes, Leil, *How to Talk to Anyone*, HarperCollins, 1999.

quotations

Many thanks to the following sources for quotations: www.brainyquote.com, www.creativequotations.com, www.quotationspage.com, www.thinkexist.com, www.wikiquote.org and www.wwnorton.com.